The Ten Minute Sexual Solution

A Busy Couple's Guide to Having More Fun, Intimacy, and Sex

Dr. Darcy Luadzers

HATHERLEIGH PRESS

NEW YORK • LONDON

Hatherleigh Press
5-22 46th Ave, Suite 200
Long Island City, NY, 11101
www.hatherleighpress.com

Library of Congress Cataloging-in-Publication Data

Luadzers, Darcy.
The ten minute sexual solution : a busy couple's guide to having more fun, intimacy, and sex / Darcy Luadzers.
    p. cm.
 ISBN 1-57826-236-4
 1. Sex instruction. 2. Sex. 3. Sexual excitement. 4. Man-woman relationships. I. Title.
  HQ31.L863 2007
  613.9'6--dc22

                         2006036582
ISBN-13: 978-1-57826-236-6
ISBN-10: 1-57826-236-4

The names identifying the characteristics of clients and clinical cases have been altered to protect confidentiality. *The Ten Minute Sexual Solution* is not intended to replace professional health care or medical advice.

The Ten Minute Sexual Solution is available for bulk purchase, special promotions, and premiums. For information on reselling and special purchase opportunities, call 1-800-528-2550 and ask for the Special Sales Manager.

Interior design by Deborah Miller, Jasmine Cardoza, Allison Furrer
Cover design by Dede Cummings

10 9 8 7 6 5 4 3 2 1
Printed in the United States

Dedication

To my husband, Dr. Jack, the other half of our "Paradox," who helped invent the Ten Minute Sexual Solution, and our five children, Stephen, Dustin, Katie, Patrick, and Zack, the mothers of invention.

Table of Contents

1 The Sexless Relationship   1

2 Sexual Power Struggles   20

3 A Guide to *The Ten Minute Sexual Solution*   45

4 Secrets of Sexual Communication   65

5 Beyond the Bedroom: What Really Makes a Relationship Work   89

6 Learn to Fight Right: Stop Arguing and Start Making Love   108

7 Maintenance Sex for Busy Couples   136

8 Creating Sexual Desire   158

9 Ten Minutes a Day: For Women   177

10 Ten Minutes a Day: For Men   213

A Closing Note from Dr. Darcy   239

Resources   241

Index   245

1

The Sexless Relationship

Sexual passion disappears even in the most loving relationships when, unexpectedly, life speeds up and steals intimate moments away. Gradually, but suddenly, half of all couples experience a shift from intimate closeness to distance as sexual passion and emotional connections fade or disappear in busy couple's lives. *The Ten Minute Sexual Solution* was written to help couples who are dissatisfied with their intimate and sexual relationship, or who would simply like to share greater sexual passion, even if they feel too busy to have the time and energy to change the most intimate part of their lives: their sex life!

Would you like to change your sex life in 30 days? Do you have 10 minutes a day for love and sexual play? What makes it worth your time to make time for love? Some people are likely to say: Anything, anywhere, anytime, anyway, you name it! But that isn't always true. Some people are likely to say: If sex only lasts 10 minutes, then I'm not going to get anything out of it! But that isn't always true, either. In just 10 minutes, couples can rekindle emotional intimacy, sexual desire, and sexual connections. We are living in a busy world that needs a fresh and different approach to intimacy and passion: one that is faster, easier, brings a pleasurable profit, but is less taxing! It's called the Ten Minute Sexual Solution, and it can help you change your relationship and sex life in one month!

The Ten Minute Sexual Solution paves a pathway to love with renewed intimacy, teaches a simple solution for sexual communication, launches a new approach to create sexual desire, and introduces maintenance sex, an innovative new way to think about and experience your relationship and sexuality. You can learn how to easily share sexual communication, including how to develop your sexual voice. Is having a sexual voice a new concept to you? You will learn about the importance of sharing yourself, sexually speaking. Most couples grow distant emotionally and physically when their sexual lives change, including talking, touch, and affection. *The Ten Minute Sexual Solution* shows you how to become close again, be friends again, and regain the emotional intimacy you've lost. For couples with conflicts, you will learn how to fight right! Anger poisons sexual desire. Learning to fight right and resolving relationship conflicts that end up in the bedroom will help you start making love again. Finally, you can find out how to create 10 minutes of maintenance sex to increase your sexual frequency and satisfaction. The Ten Minute Sexual Solution takes just 10 minutes a day to deepen your emotional intimacy and change your sex life forever.

WHO NEEDS *THE TEN MINUTE SEXUAL SOLUTION?*

Every day, couples come into my sex therapy office, worried about their relationship or marriage, wondering what happened to their passionate love life and if they can ever get it back. Most couples are never taught about and don't know how to be lovers over time in a long-term relationship, or to manage sexual differences as they each grow and life changes. Many people doubt that they can find a common sexual ground when they seem so far apart in their relationship. Hope lies in understanding your sexual differences and creating new intimate connections using a 10 minute sexual solution that helps couples make time to make love.

Almost every couple in a long-term relationship or marriage needs to have a loving solution for taking care of each partner's emotional and sexual needs over time. At the beginning of a relationship, almost all couples seem to be sexually compatible. They seem to make love all the time! There's not a whole lot of difference in sexual needs then. You don't worry over whether or not you're going to make love, or when or where you're going to have sex, since you're figuring out a way to do it all the time, right? But over time, individuals' true sexual natures emerge and evolve—months and years after commitments or marriage vows have been taken. Sexual drive can change over time, for either partner, for many physical and psychological reasons. When sex changes, changes in emotional intimacy follow. Or, more typically, when the emotional relationship changes, sex changes. Understanding those reasons, and coping with life's stresses, is the motivation for *The Ten Minute Sexual Solution*.

> ## Sometimes, over time, couples begin to feel and act more like roommates rather than lovers.

The number one reason people say they don't have enough sex is because they are too busy or too exhausted for sex. Many people wait to have sex until "the time is right." For many couples, living real lives, with real jobs and perfectly imperfect relationships, with in-laws and kids and pets and parents, houses and spouses and mortgages and high rents, finding the time for sex and even thinking about sex is a big problem.

> ## Life speeds up and steals intimate moments away.

Couples often don't find the time to think about sex, want or desire sex, let alone have enough time to make love. The ideals of romance might include a week-long vacation alone, spending Saturday in bed until noon, or sharing quiet time together to light candles, drink wine, and laugh. Yet, if you have to wait until the ideal situation on your annual vacation to spend the day together, when you're relaxed, totally focused on each other, with leisure time to kill, it's going to be a very long year waiting, right? What happened to the passionate, romantic, sexy hours of lovemaking from your dating years? Or when you were first married? Or the "endless opportunities" that living together every day would allow you to share?

> ### Life happened!

Sex often becomes the lowest priority for couples after work, friends, children, church, family obligations, and other important interests or obligations. So, in the meantime, while you are waiting for a luxurious weekend vacation day to have time and energy for passionate intimate moments, you need a new solution to find the time to connect as a couple, emotionally and sexually.

While couples say they "don't have time for sex," the truth is that they don't have the habits to make love happen.

Couples can learn a new way of life to share love, become emotionally close, discover the time and new skills to communicate about sex, create sexual desire, and make love, too. The Ten Minute Sexual Solution helps couples create moments for intimacy and sexual passion in 10 minutes a day!

THE REALITY OF SEXLESS RELATIONSHIPS

A sexless relationship is clinically defined as having sexual intercourse less than 10 times a year, or never. Astonishingly, it is estimated that 20 percent of all married couples have a sexless marriage and 30 percent of non-married couples have a sexless relationship, meaning millions of couples are living in low-sex or sexless relationships. About half of long-term couples have sex less than once a week, and many people are saddened by their lost sexual passion. One important survey[1] on married couples found:

- 33 percent of couples did not have sex in the last month
- 15 percent of couples had sex "a few times a year or not at all"
- 45 percent of couples reported having sex "a few times a month"

Some couples agree that sex once or twice a month or less is okay for their relationship, perhaps due to a compatibility of sexual desires. But for at least 50 percent of people, at some point in their relationships, low sexual frequency is a very big problem! For the 60 percent of couples who have sex less than once a week, when one person in the relationship would like to have sex a few times a week, sexual incompatibility can be a major dissatisfaction in their relationship for both partners. A sexual impasse can result, causing conflicts and fights, and leaving partners feeling frustrated or defeated, both sexually and emotionally.

Couples are often out of sexual sync for many different reasons, including their busy lives, their inability to talk openly about sex, and differences in sexual desire. A couple's entire relationship can shift when they are faced with sexual differences or when one partner has a lower sexual desire than the other. Some couples slowly withdraw from each other, touching less, kissing less passionately, and fighting more than they make love. Some people think their partner no longer wants them, when often it's not a personal or sexual rejection, but a lack of knowing how to handle sexual differences, sexual change, or how to maintain an intimate relationship when sex changes. If you are in a relationship where intimacy and passion has faded, you are not alone. *The Ten Minute Sexual Solution* was written for you.

At least half of all couples need a sexual solution to bridge differences in desire for sex over the course of their relationship, while balancing their busy lives.

SEXUAL COMMUNICATION AND INTIMACY

Making the Ten Minute Sexual Solution work for you as a busy couple requires building an emotional foundation for your relationship on which you can create a sexual relationship. First, you will learn the secrets of sexual communication, to learn to how to talk about sex, or any sensitive topic, to strengthen and deepen intimacy as a couple. It is amazing to me, as a sex therapist, how little some couples actually talk about their sex life, or how uncomfortable they feel just saying sexual words with each other. Learning to simply discuss sexuality is the beginning of essential sexual communication. Second, sexual communication is key to developing emotional intimacy and negotiating change in your relationship outside the bedroom, so you both will want to share more physical intimacy.

"WE DON'T EVEN SEE EACH OTHER ALONE ANYMORE!"

Many couples barely take the time to sit and talk or spend time having fun together, let alone having sex. Most people spend more time with their coworkers or computers than with their lovers or partners. Some people are busy with their jobs, children, and outside activities. Sometimes couples just don't know how to balance life with their love life. Some people are avoiding each other because of resentments and anger.

Couples who share greater intimacy often feel like making love more. Can you imagine having sex first, then maybe dating? That is what is happening inside some relationships and marriages, with people wondering, "Why doesn't my partner want to have sex?" Women often say they want to be made love to outside the bedroom before they want to go into the bedroom. Many people say they'd like to feel sensuous and seductive, but they don't take the time to share that with each other anymore. You can learn to create transitions from life to your love life to become a loving couple again, creating more desire to share lovemaking. Learning to take just a little time for your relationship will help you rekindle and maintain a loving relationship. In 10 minutes a day, you can renew your emotional relationship and find time for a sexual relationship, even if it's just maintenance sex.

WHAT IS MAINTENANCE SEX?

Imagine the possibility of sexual synchronicity. Maintenance sex is real sex for busy couples and a part of the Ten Minute Sexual Solution that will help you change your sex life. It is a very special way of sharing sexuality together as a couple: a very quick and easy sexual solution to increase your sexual frequency and forge a special sexual bond. Couples can learn to be loving partners with each other for life within the freedom of monogamy and to love each other in a very special, caring way!

In many couple's busy lives, sex comes last. Couples maintain their lawns, their cars, their pensions, their jobs, their plants, their homes, their pets, and spend a lot more than 10 minutes a day doing it.

> **Maintenance sex is taking 10 minutes to focus on fulfilling one or both partner's basic sexual needs, until you have an opportunity for longer lasting lovemaking moments.**

Couple's sexual desires are often out of sync. Maintenance sex can help bridge the differences and difficulties in timing needed to give each other sexual attention and sexual care on a regular basis. Maintenance sex is a way to create high quality quickies for couples who care about each other. However, maintenance sex is not just about having sexual intercourse; it is about creating different kinds of sexual moments that are playful, flexible, and mutually acceptable. Creating new sexual scripts that are only limited by your imagination is possible. Permission and encouragement can create endless opportunities for new sexual scenarios. Chapter 7 describes the details of maintenance sex and its role in your relationship. Creating a relationship that has a foundation upon which to experience more frequent sexual encounters, and how to negotiate and plan for hot, sometimes passionate, sometimes simply satisfying 10 minute interludes of sex that accommodate each other's basic sexual desires is part of the Ten Minute Sexual Solution.

SEXUAL DESIRE: THE SEXLESS STRUGGLE

A major reason why couples have sexless relationships is a lack of sexual desire. One third (33 percent) of women and 13 percent of men report having low sexual desire which results in low sexual frequency for many couples[2]. The truth about sexless relationships is that couples typically only have sex as often as the person with the lowest sexual desire wants sex, which may not be very often. Differences in sexual desire are common in long-term relationships. Often couples have one partner with higher sexual desire and one with lower sexual desire. Sexual desire differences can range from simple to complex, situational or long-term, but a difference in sexual desire is the most common reason why couples experience deep dissatisfaction in sexual frequency and have sexual struggles.

Sexual conflicts can turn into power struggles that change a couple's overall relationship and can even destroy the emotional bond and love between two people. The tension over sex affects affection, as well: People with lower sexual desires avoid intimate touch, even hugging and cuddling, to avoid any physical contact that might lead to sex. Chapter 2 discusses sexual power struggles that are common in couples with sexual desire differences, and teaches how to avoid or change these in your relationship. Some couples give up and stop having sex, settling on a sexless relationship, which is a tragedy. Before you give up on your sex life, let me introduce to you new approaches to understanding and creating sexual desire that may change your relationship and life.

The Ten Minute Sexual Solution helps couples who have sexual differences and will help you get your intimate and passionate life back on track, regardless of the reason. Because many couples face differences in sexual desire that often affect the core of their relationship, this book addresses the sexual matters and very special circumstances of both the higher and lower desire partners. Each of your concerns is important in your relationship. Each of you has specific emotional and sexual issues that need to be addressed if your relationship is going to change. Each of you deserves to have a voice, to be heard, to be understood, and to understand how this book can work for you individually. Let me introduce the *The Ten Minute Sexual Solution* to each of you.

JUST FOR YOU: TO THE LOWER-DESIRE PARTNER

First of all, did you know that you can have lower sexual desire than your partner and still be sexually "normal"? Very few couples are completely sexually compatible! Even when couples share similar desires for sex, they can be sexually out of sync, wanting to share sexual connections at different times, for different reasons, and in different ways. The truth is, you may have normal sexual desire, not low sexual desire, but as a couple you may simply have different sexual desires. When one partner has lower sexual desire than the other, you will have a sexual compatibility gap. Unfortunately, the wider your sexual desire gap, the more likely you will have sexual struggles, which *The Ten Minute Sexual Solution* will help you learn to manage better as a couple.

While "normal sexual desire" is difficult to define, if you desire sex less than once or twice a month, or your sexual desire has greatly decreased, most sex therapists will agree that you have low or inhibited sexual desire, which is discussed in chapter 2. Some of the reasons for low sexual desire are very simple, some complex.

Amazingly, some of the solutions to changing low sexual desire are much easier than most people can imagine; however, if your problem has been ongoing for a long time, your relationship may have already experienced many negative changes, such as repeated sexual conflicts and sexual avoidance, and you may feel it is impossible to change your relationship or sexual self now.

If you have inhibited or low sexual desire, you may have an individual problem, but it may also be related to problems in your relationship or stressful situations in your life. This book will help you learn about sexual desire, understand many of the causes of low sexual desire, and unravel the complicated consequences of different sexual desires in your relationship. Unlike other books that may focus on *your* problem of low sexual desire, this book will help you identify and understand low sexual desire both individually and as a couple, identifying and solving the various problems that lead to low sexual desire, and providing sexual solutions for your situation as a couple.

The sad fact is that the partner with the lower sexual desire is often targeted as the cause of a couple's sexual problem. Often the lower-desire partner is blamed for the sexual problems, which may lead to feelings of sexually inadequacy. Here are some statements that come straight from my couch as a sex therapist.

- I feel so pressured to have sex that now I HATE sex!
- Maybe I'm just not a sexual person!
- Sex feels like a duty, not a desire.
- I don't know if anyone can understand ME: I just don't want to have sex.
- I understand that my partner wants and needs more sex, and I feel guilty that I avoid him. I don't want to get divorced, but I don't know what else to do.
- What's wrong with me? I want to want sex!
- I used to like sex, but now I don't even have the time or energy to think about it.

- Maybe my partner is a sex addict and there's something wrong with HER! Even when we have sex, it is never enough.

All of these different feelings, thoughts, and fears will be addressed in this book. Interestingly, the most common cause of low sexual desire has nothing to do with an individual's sexual desire at all—it has to do with anger in a relationship. As hard as it might be for your higher desire partner to understand, some people actually don't want to have sex when they are mad at their partner! The angry, distant partner is often blamed as having a sexual problem, when in fact resentments and relationship problems are killing sexual desire. If you once felt passion and desire, it is possible that there is nothing physically wrong with you, as it is normal to lose sexual desire in the face of anger. Chapter 6 is aimed at helping couples learn to fight right, so they can resolve resentments, remove anger, and allow people to feel loving feelings toward each other, including the rekindling of sexual desire.

There are many reasons for low sexual desire besides relationship conflicts that end up in the bedroom. Two of the top reasons are sexual pain and not experiencing sexual pleasure, which are very important to address prior to working on your relationship with your partner.

Did you know that 75 percent of men and only 29 percent of women ALWAYS have orgasms during sex?[3]

It seems more NORMAL to NOT desire sex, if you don't get much out of sex! If it were NORMAL to always have orgasms, maybe more women would have NORMAL sexual desire!

For some people, learning how to experience greater sexual pleasure will help create sexual desire. Most sex therapists, most pop psychology books, and magazines that share "new sexual secrets" (especially targeted at women) teach people that if they learn about their bodies and learn to have orgasms then they will want to have sex. Right? Yes, this is true for some women, so chapter 9 teaches women how to have more reliable and frequent orgasms. Yet, some women do have sexual pleasure and experience orgasms, but they *still* do not feel sexual desire or think about sex and want sex. This book includes several sections to help both men and women with low sexual desire understand their sexual selves, learn how to experience sexual pleasure, and create sexual desire. The truth is many people, both men and women, have sexual desire, but they experience it in a different way than most people currently understand.

This book will introduce you to a new way of thinking about how some people experience sexual feelings. Some individuals need to experience physical touch, including cuddling, caressing, kissing, and sexual touch first, and then they experience sexual excitement, with sexual desire *following* the feelings of sexual arousal. For some people, if they delay or avoid sex until they feel desire, they will seldom want sex, even though when they do have sex, they can enjoy it. This new approach to sex, discussed in chapter 8, will help many people understand themselves and experience their sexuality more fully!

> Some people need to experience sexual feelings first,
> then they feel sexual desire.
> Sometimes people don't experience a feeling
> until they're feeling the experience.

These truths are an introduction to a whole new idea, a different paradigm, and a shift in thinking about sexual desire that can change your sexual relationship. Many women don't think about sex very often, and they don't have as many sexual fantasies; they don't desire sex as often as men. Yet, for many women, the truth is that once they get sexually excited, many women feel desire, love sex as much as men, and can run circles around them sexually! The old approach to low sexual desire was to focus on trying to increase a person's desire or interest in sex. This book introduces a new approach to understanding and creating sexual desire in chapter 8. Chapter 2 also reveals common causes of and therapy for individuals with a low sexual desire. For the lower-desire partner: Allow yourself to imagine changing what you have learned about how sex happens, feeling sexual desire, wanting your lover, embracing your lover wanting you, and consider the possibility of being a person who makes love more often, and enjoys it!

For some individuals, sexual desire can be a very complex sexual problem that may be beyond the scope of this book. If you have experienced past sexual trauma or have other sexual dysfunctions, you may wish to seek a professional consultation with a sex therapist individually, prior to working on your sexual relationship as a couple. As a sex therapist, I strongly recommend not engaging in sex that causes unwanted pain; seek to resolve this problem first. If you do have physical sexual pain, I recommend reading the second half of chapter 2, which explains a little known common cause of sexual pain and discomfort. However, if you feel very strongly against wanting to read this book or trying to change your sexual relationship, if you feel averse to sex, or even extremely embarrassed about talking about sex with your partner, you may need to seek professional help from a sex therapist (see aasect.org for one in your area), rather than proceed with sexual self-help or *The Ten Minute Sexual Solution*.

JUST FOR YOU: TO THE HIGHER-DESIRE PARTNER

Often the higher-desire partner is the one trying to figure out what happened to his or her sex life. You might be the person reading articles, surfing the Internet, looking for books, making suggestions for change in your relationship, and trying to change your sexual relationship. The higher-desire partner's true feelings and needs are often neglected in research, magazine articles, and media portrayals on sexually discrepant relationships. You are sometimes depicted as sex starved, sex addicted, nymphomaniacs, or sex-crazed individuals who can "never get enough." In my sex therapy practice, often the higher-desire partners are incredibly patient, compassionate, and empathetic, but may feel sad, sexually frustrated, and desperate for an answer to a sexual enigma. Some people describe feeling heartbreaking disappointment over their sexless relationship or marriage. This book was written to help you, as well as your partner, understand what is happening in your relationship and with your sex life, and to provide a sexual solution that can really make a difference in your life, for the rest of your life!

Sometimes, you may blame your partner for the lack of sex, since your partner is rejecting your sexual advances, avoiding you physically, and not initiating sex. But lower-desire partners may never initiate sex because they "never get a chance!" You are already asking them for sex again before they get a chance to think about sex again! Sometimes the higher-desire partner will wait until they are approached for sex, counting the days, weeks, or months between sexual liaisons, feeling angry and trying to find out how long it will be until their partner initiates sex. Over time, even higher-desire partners will often stop initiating sex because they get hurt or tired of being rejected, feeling unwanted, or just knowing their partners doesn't want sex very often.

In the long-run, higher-desire partners can blame themselves for the sexual rejection, fearing they are no longer attractive or sexually inadequate, and wondering what is going on that they are living in a seemingly sexless relationship. Here are some statements that come straight from my couch as a sex therapist.

- What is wrong with me that my partner does not want me?
- Am I no longer attractive to her?
- Why aren't I enough for him?
- Why doesn't he want to have sex?
- Does she still love me?
- Is our relationship in trouble?
- Are we going to get divorced?
- Is my partner gay?
- Is my partner having an affair?
- The only way we'll have sex is if I put on the pressure or guilt or make demands
- Will I have to live in a sexless marriage? I can't live this way!

These feelings, assumptions, and fears resulting from low sexual frequency are very painful for the higher-desire partner. Yet in many cases, lower sexual frequency is not a result of any of these emotional fears or realities in a relationship. Often couples who love each other and are attracted to each other still have infrequent sex or sexless relationships. Often sexless relationships are not a result of two people not loving each other or wanting each other, but simply the result of a difference in sexual desire! Learning to understand and manage sexual differences, including reasons why your partner has a lower sexual desire, is a part of the Ten Minute Sexual Solution!

Sadly, when your partner desires sex less than you, changes can occur outside your sexual relationship as well. A shift in your relationship happens, where it can seem as if you change from being lovers to being roommates. If your partner has a lower sexual desire, he or she will often avoid physical touch, affection, and kissing, because they are afraid it will lead to sex. Your passionate, playful, fun relationship has turned into two separate people who sit on different sides of the couch or surf on separate computers, watch TV in different rooms or sleep in different beds, and share little beyond the shallow details of daily life. When relationships change, many people give up hope of having a close, loving, and intimate relationship again. Learning to become friends and lovers again, and avoiding distance in your relationship, is possible.

Many higher-desire partners resort to repeatedly making demands for sex and won't take no for an answer. Demands may involve pleading, yelling, unwanted touch, starting fights, or making threats. Sometimes it is not just because you want to have sex, but because you want to be wanted. Yet sexual control is an illusion that creates a sexual crisis a relationship. Paradoxically, sexual coercion has long-term side effects of destroying love, desire, and sexual pleasure, and can affect an entire relationship.

Working the steps of the Ten Minute Sexual Solution, you will have an opportunity to learn to communicate effectively with your partner, to uncover and understand your sexual differences. You will learn many new approaches and explanations to grasp and solve your sexual problem. Rather than blaming your partner or yourself for your relationship or sexual problems, you can uncover the roots of your problems as a couple. Begin by working on being friends, improving your emotional relationship and closeness, resolving any relationship fights or conflicts, and opening your mind to innovative sexual solutions for your relationship.

Throughout this book, you will find professional sex therapy advice on improving your relationship and sex life, to advise both you and your partner on how to get your intimate and passionate relationship back on track. One of the areas that you as a higher-desire person will need to address before you can work on your relationship as a partnership is any of your individual problems that may be causing conflicts or anger in your relationship. One of the major reasons for lower sexual desire is anger rooted in relationship conflicts. For example, many couples harbor resentment over conflicts in the division of domestic duties. Unmet expectations or a lack of agreement over expectations can lead to resentments, broken trust, and decreased sexual desire. In addition, if you are having any major life problems, such as addictions, chronic work problems, depression, anger management problems, a medical condition, or affairs, you may need professional help to resolve those problems first. If either of you has a major life problem, get the help you need or make a commitment to individual change, so you can work with each other to regain trust and create a new foundation for an intimate and sexual relationship.

A NOTE FOR COUPLES

The Ten Minute Sexual Solution was written for YOU. I believe that most couples can experience sexual passion, increased emotional intimacy, and sexual magic. Most people come to sex therapy feeling very uncomfortable talking about sexuality, and nervous about sharing their intimate lives with a stranger. One of the benefits of sex therapy is to begin a dialog about sex, between the two of you. *The Ten Minute Sexual Solution* is a sex therapy guide for couples in long-term relationships who wish to begin this dialog on their own, a journey that can change your sex lives for the rest of your lives. Sexual passion is possible, working at it just 10 minutes a day!

The Ten Minute Sexual Solution is written for couples in long-term committed monogamous relationships, whether you are married or not. Some sections of this book refer to marriage, but these sections are not intended to exclude those committed couples that are not "legally married." For ease of writing, a conventional approach is used at times, using he/she pronouns and heterosexual relationship references, to avoid duplication in jargon (he/he and she/she). This is not intended to exclude or offend couples in same-sex relationships, who face many of the same sexual struggles as heterosexual couples. In some examples, same-sex couples' stories are shared, not intending to exclude or offend heterosexual couples, but to represent the broad spectrum of couples that seek sexual solutions in their relationships.

The Ten Minute Sexual Solution addresses *people* who have relationship and sexual problems, including different male and female perspectives of higher and lower sexual desire. More frequently women have low or lower sexual desire than their partners, while more men are the higher-desire partner. Since a majority of couples consist of male higher-desire/female lower-desire, some sections of this book refer to the lower-desire partner as female, and the higher-desire partner as male, for ease of writing and to avoid duplication. This is not intended to exclude couples who are female higher-desire/male lower-desire or same-sex couples. Often these couples have very similar relationship issues and dynamics in reverse, although there are some gender differences in their relationship dynamics. Chapters 9 and 10 both include information just for the higher-desire female and lower-desire male. Couples in same-sex relationships have problems with discrepant desire as well, and many of the components of *The Ten Minute Sexual Solution* can be applied to most higher-/lower-desire couples, regardless of gender or sexual preference.

The Ten Minute Sexual Solution is a new and powerful approach to help busy couples set a foundation for a more passionate and intimate relationship, including sharing a more satisfying sexual relationship. This book can help you learn to handle the normal, natural differences that couples have with sexual timing and differences, as well as learn to manage differences in sexual desire. *The Ten Minute Sexual Solution* is not intended to replace sex therapy for couples who need to have professional help; however, it is a guide for many couples who would love to learn how to change their relationship and rediscover the sexual magic in their life.

So welcome to *The Ten Minute Sexual Solution*, an innovative approach to help couples become lovers, more often, again. Open your mind to a new sexuality for real couples.

- Ten minute solutions for sexual communication
- Ten minute tips for renewing intimacy
- Ten minute solutions to create sexual desire
- Ten minute maintenance sex solutions
- Ten steps to stop fighting and start making love

No matter how busy you are, how many hours of housework or work you do outside the home, how many kids or in-laws or pets you care for, whether you are gay or straight, fat or thin, young or old, male or female, married or not, many people with sexless relationships can learn new sexual solutions to change their sex lives by working at it just 10 minutes a day. Good luck on your sexual journey!

CHAPTER

2

Sexual Power Struggles

Sexual power struggles change a couple's relationship. Differences in sexual desire can create very complex relationship problems that often result in sexual power struggles. Some power struggles are very destructive, some simply sad. Happy couples, loving people, good people, individuals who once laughed, loved, and shared a wonderful relationship change, often gradually over time. Gradually, but suddenly, ordinary people find themselves in a relationship that feels strange or even bizarre when they look at how they relate to each other and treat each other on a daily basis. Sexual secrets and shame are created that seemingly no one can understand, especially the individuals themselves.

Loving partners that once treated each other with admiration and respect can sink to lows of anger, anxiety, and embarrassment, feeling alone in their silent suffering, their sexless relationship, their sexual struggle. Couples often cling to their love, secretly holding the reality of their relationship together under the power of the vows of marriage or commitment. Rather than wondering how long you can hold on, this chapter will help you begin to hold on to hope, through understanding instead. Couples often don't understand or do not cope with sexual differences very well. Very few people are taught how to manage differences in sexual desire. This chapter will explain different ways that couples handle sexual differences, including the destructive relationship patterns that commonly result from handling sexual differences with blame, fear, confusion, and intimidation. The second half of this chapter will introduce basic information to begin understanding low sexual desire, including some important but simple solutions for changing sexual desire that couple need to know prior to beginning the Ten Minute Sexual Solution.

PART I: SEXUAL POWER STRUGGLES OVER DIFFERENT SEXUAL DESIRES

Many couples experience tragic consequences in their relationship over sexual power struggles, due to one partner having lower sexual desire or individual differences in sexual desires. Yet, many relationship problems are not simply due to sexual desire differences; they result from a power struggle on the emotional bond and love between two people. Couples experience a shift, a gradual movement away from each other, both emotionally and physically. People avoid each other, not touching each other. Silence takes over the night, in bed. People ask themselves: How did we get this way? Why do we treat each other so badly at times? What are we going to do?

> **Regardless of the reason, couples who have differences in sexual desire often develop dysfunctional relationships, with power struggles that can destroy their love.**

SEXUAL DIFFERENCES

Partners often have differences in sexual desire simply because they are different people. Even when couples have similar sexual desires, couples are often sexually out of sync depending on when and how they want to share sexual interactions. Sometimes the difference is due to an individual's feelings on any given day, depending on his or her career, medical or mental health, responsibilities with children or parents, house and car maintenance, or menstrual cycle. Over time, most couples find that one person in their relationship has a higher sexual desire than their partner, and one partner has a lower sexual desire. Over the course of a relationship or marriage, this can also change. In long-term relationships, understanding and handling this difference is essential to couples having a satisfying sexual relationship.

> Managing a long-term sexual relationship is very different than dating. To start, couples need to understand and learn about different sexual desires.

Differences in sexual desire, for whatever reasons on any given day, week, or year, result in people not being sexually matched at that time. Rather than focusing right now on the reasons or blaming each other for the causes of sexual differences, consider the simple reality that people want different amounts of sexual activity. Often the problem of sexual differences is a nuts and bolts equation. If there are 10 nuts and only 2 bolts, you will only get 2 matches. Let's consider the case of "Sam and Jo." If Sam wants sex 10 times and Jo wants sex 2 times (a week or month or year), they will likely only have sex 2 times. In reality, Sam gets to have sex anytime that Jo will agree to it. Jo controls sex. Jo may not even want to control sex! Often, it's not a power game. It's a mathematical reality, because one person wants less sex. With few exceptions, the truth is that the person with the lowest desire for sexual frequency will control how often a couple has sex.

> **The secret truth is that the lower-desire partner will control sex, whether they want to or not.**

Every couple has basically four different ways to manage sexual differences in a long-term relationship. A couple has choices of how to handle one person having lower sexual desire, which often happens in a sexual relationship. A couple can be accepting of the lower desire and have less frequent sex, or the couple can be nonaccepting. An individual may choose to be sexually accommodating and have sex with his partner, even if he really doesn't feel any sexual desire at the time, or she can choose to not be sexually accommodating and not engage in sex.

FOUR WAYS COUPLES HANDLE SEXUAL DESIRE DIFFERENCES

1. Acceptance of lower sexual desire and low sexual frequency.
2. Acceptance of lower sexual desire, but the lower-desire partner is sexually accommodating, with mutual consent.
3. Nonacceptance of lower sexual desire and lower-desire partner is sexually accommodating, but with resentment and anger.
4. Nonacceptance of lower sexual desire and one partner is not sexually accommodating, but the higher-desire partner uses sexual coercion and sexual badgering to control sex.

Couples choose how to manage differences in sexual desire in several different ways, often without thinking about why they do it or if they have other choices. Couples often become entrenched in the way they choose to handle their sexual differences, despite many choices. With the first option, the higher-desire partners are often sexually dissatisfied, since they have low sexual frequency, and the lower-desire partners may feel pressured or guilty. Some couples manage to learn to live with it, but in some cases, an unsatisfied partner may grow emotionally distant with resentment, become vulnerable to having affairs, or divorce. With options three and four, the lower-desire partner may learn to live with an unwanted higher sexual frequency, but over time, a lack of mutual agreement or consent will lead to resentments, sexual dysfunctions, and serious relationship problems.

The truth is that the options for handling sexual differences other than option two lead to problems within a relationship. With differences in desire, the goal is for couples to choose and use option two: acceptance of lower sexual desire, using sexual accommodation with mutual consent—and in most cases, loving agreement—to handle sexual differences. For partners that are not in loving agreement now, hope for sexual change lies in working together as a couple to change the way you handle your differences in sexual desire. Of course, some individuals may change and increase their sexual desire, but when there is a difference, making agreements to manage this difference together as a couple can lead to a more satisfying sexual relationship.

The fourth option (nonacceptance, no sexual accommodation, and sexual coercion) is commonly seen in couples and sex therapy. In many cases, the higher-desire partners, fueled by sexual frustration and emotional fears about themselves and their relationships, revert to control and use sexual coercion or sexual badgering to reverse the control of sex. Many couples have experienced this power struggle with their relationship, at least on a rare occasion; hence, the following sections describe the negative effects of sexual power struggles on a relationship.

FEARS IN A SEXLESS RELATIONSHIP

It can be difficult for higher-partners to understand why they are not having more sex, especially when it is quite infrequent. It can be emotionally devastating to feel that you are not wanted by your partner, with whom you love and crave to share physical love. Being rejected sexually often translates into emotional fears and false assumptions about why you have a sexless relationship. So often, so sadly, higher-desire partners blame themselves, fear they are no longer attractive, and wonder what is wrong with their relationships. Or they blame their partners, wondering if their partners are gay, having an affair, or have psychological or sexual problems.

These feelings and false assumptions resulting from low sexual frequency are emotional torture! In many cases, lower sexual frequency is not a result of any of these emotional fears or realities in a relationship. Really! Many people need to stop torturing themselves with fears and insecurities that are hurting them, but are not based on the truth. Often partners who love each other and are attracted to each other still have different sexual desires. Yet, when higher-desire partners have fears about themselves and their relationship, they might resort to handling their sexual differences with option four, or sexual coercion to reverse the control of sex. Here is where a sexual power struggle can become destructive.

SEXUAL COERCION AND SEXUAL BADGERING

Using "Sam and Jo" as an example of this situation, you can see how a couple can become entangled in a sexual power struggle, which is so important to understand and change.

Sam wants or demands sex several times a week and Jo goes along with it, even though she doesn't want it. Sam has a lot of power in the relationship, and Jo has sex with Sam even when Jo doesn't desire sex. For example, Sam might say or communicate through behavior, "If we don't have sex more often, then _____." Fill in the blank with a meaningful threat, and Sam wins in the short run, while in the long run Jo's sexual desire will continue to diminish because of resentment and anger toward Sam. The blank may be filled in with:

- I'll divorce you.
- I'll pout or brood.
- I won't give you any money.
- I'll walk around angry until we have sex.
- I'll have an affair.

- I'll break it off with you and take our children away.
- I'll tell everyone you're frigid.
- I'll fight with you about sex and remind you of all your faults.
- I'll fight with you about everything but sex, but it will actually be about sex.

Sexual badgering is when the higher-desire partner repeatedly makes demands for sex and won't take no for an answer. Demands may involve pleading, yelling, unwanted touching, pawing or groping, starting fights, making threats, or not leaving a partner alone after repeated requests to do so. Sexual coercion may not be verbal badgering, but lower-desire partners feel sexual pressure because she knows her partner wants sex by the way he acts, such as brooding, being in a bad mood, or being emotionally and physically distant for no reason, filling the air with tension. Some people feel sexual pressure because of their beliefs and guilt about sex and their changed sexual relationship—not due to how their partners really feel, but because they've never talked about it.

> **Sexual badgering has long-term side effects of destroying love, desire, and sexual pleasure, and even destroying a relationship or marriage.**

Sexual badgering and coercion are often causes of sexual shame, as the higher-desire person often feels embarrassed or bad for engaging in this behavior. Recipients of sexual badgering also feel sexual shame for participating in this power struggle. Often the lower-desire person in this situation feels very sexually inadequate and can even feel victimized in extreme cases.

THE CYCLE OF SEXUAL POWER STRUGGLES

A cycle of sexual power struggles begins. First, there is a low sexual frequency, which varies depending on the individuals' sexual desire and the gap of sexual needs. The higher-desire partners badger or coerce the lower-desire partners into having sex. The lower-desire partners give in and have sex when they don't want to, sometimes just to go to sleep at night, sometimes to change their partners' bad moods, sometimes to avoid a threat. The lower-desire partners know if they have sex, they'll finally be left alone and avoid real or perceived threats. After sex, the lower-desire partners might feel relieved for a couple of days or so, but then they know or fear sexual demands or coercion will begin again; resentment sets in, and they start to avoid sex, again. Lower-desire partners might avoid sex or become defensive or passive-aggressive, which is discussed below, in reaction to fears that they'll soon face more sexual demands, starting the cycle over again. Sadly, victims of sexual badgering often lose all feelings of sexual desire for their partner, since coercion has a killer effect on natural sexual desire, which only fuels the cycle of a sexual power struggle.

> **Sexual coercion often works in the short run, but in the long run it kills sexual desire, fueling more sexual power struggles.**

Higher-desire partners may feel sexual relief or emotional reassurance that their partners want them after they share sex. Yet sometimes they feel very dissatisfied if they know or sense their partners are not willing participants or did not enjoy sex. If they do not feel sexually reassured, they may demand more sex, or more from sex. Higher-desire partners might complain about lifeless or boring sex, wanting their partners to "get into it," or have an orgasm, to prove they are loved by their partners or to prove to lower-desire partners that sex is enjoyable, so they might want sex more. Both men and women fake orgasms and fake sexual enjoyment to avoid these complaints, which puts more pressure on sex to be a performance rather than an act of pleasure and sharing of love.

SEXUAL SELF-DEFENSE AND SEXUAL PASSIVE-AGGRESSIVENESS

A loss of sexual desire is often an unintended by-product of sexual coercion or badgering. Some people simply shut off all of their sexual feelings, having been turned off of sex from sexual pressure. Without realizing it is happening, individuals may lose their interest in sex or label themselves as having "low sexual desire," because sex has become drudgery. A lack of sexual drive may also be self-defense against an emotionally abusive or conflicted relationship or marriage in general. Individuals may develop sexual passive-aggressive behaviors as a defense against sexual coercion or other types of emotional conflict in the relationship. Passive-aggressiveness is a behavior defined by a lack of behavior or unspoken actions that are actually hostile or unsympathetic to someone else. A passive-aggressive response to sexually controlling behavior may include simply refusing to engage in sex, avoiding sex, or acting disinterested. Acting passive by doing nothing sexually sends a strong message to a sexually controlling partner.

> For an individual with lower sexual desire, passive-aggressive behavior may arise as an important self-defense, in an attempt to maintain a sexual identity that is being destroyed by a person they love.

A victim of sexual coercion often has very interesting ways to avoid sex. In the case of Sam and Jo, Jo might find defensive ways to get around Sam's power. When someone is controlling and uncompromising, and discussion and resolution of the problem is unsuccessful or impossible, generally the only defense is a passive-aggressive form of retaliation and power that can range from mild to severe forms, from simple sexual avoidance to sexual passive-aggressiveness.

SEXUAL PASSIVE-AGGRESSIVE BEHAVIORS
• Go to bed early or late
• Sleep with the children, using various excuses

- Play or "work" on the computer all night
- Bring work home that "has to get done"
- Talk on the phone for hours to family and friends
- No longer sleep nude, "dress like a nun" in bed, refuse to wear lingerie
- Dress in a separate room or area
- Keep the kids up late, sometimes doing "urgent" homework
- Have sex, but refuse to share pleasure or have an orgasm
- Refuse to engage in a variety of different sexual acts, such as oral sex
- Gain weight, dress unkempt, or not shower or brush teeth, to become undesirable to partner and turn them off sexually
- Have an affair

Passive-aggressive sexual behaviors may be unintentional habits that individuals with lower sexual desire develop over time to avoid sexual relationships, without even realizing what they are doing. Yet some people may also be deliberately sexually passive-aggressive or even go as far as to engage in sexual "payback" to their partners. One "Jo" that I had in therapy complied completely with "Sam's" demands and had sex with Sam nearly every day they were together in their 20-year marriage. However, partly as payback and partly to enjoy her own true sexuality, she had a string of lovers on the side with whom she enjoyed lovemaking. This infidelity was a very hostile, passive-aggressive act toward her partner to override his control and retaliate against him, without ever directly resolving the "unsolvable problem." It is amazing to me to what lengths people will go to solve relationship and sexual problems in order to get what they want sexually in a relationship, instead of working together, as a team, to resolve their problems.

> **If you coerce your partner into having sex, you will set up a scenario of passive-aggression at worst, but even at best, sexual pressure is a huge turn-off that starts a self-fulfilling prophecy of a sexless relationship.**

Sexual control is an illusion that creates a sexual crisis a relationship. The solution to differences in sexual desire is not coercion or demands! Even when told this, some clients with higher desire have pleaded, "But, if I don't keep pressuring her and demanding sex... we'll never have sex!" No! It is guaranteed that you will never have *lovemaking* if you don't find a different solution to your problem.

THE TRUTH ABOUT SEXUAL POWER STRUGGLES

Sexual coercion and sexual badgering are desperate measures that people take to try to solve a problem. It is not uncommon to see this type of behavior with otherwise loving couples that have a sexual discrepancy problem. Sexual conflicts can escalate to a level of hostility or fights before a couple decides to seek help with a sex therapist. Often, a huge fight over sex is the trigger event that made people identify and realize their problem was out of control and unmanageable and that they needed help. However, sexual badgering can be emotional abuse and a red flag in a relationship. If a person will be emotionally abusive inside the bedroom, he or she may be emotionally abusive outside the bedroom, as well. People who are emotionally coercive with sex can be controlling in other ways, such as with money, criticism, and being judgmental with friends, family, jobs, or child rearing.

As with other relationship or marriage problems, a couple that has a few "kitchen fights" and loses their tempers with yelling, calling someone a name, or slamming a door is wrong, and it's inappropriate behavior. Period. A single episode or rare occasion of such behavior is, honestly, common with most couples. Transgressions, with remorse, can generally be forgiven. On the other hand, chronic emotional abuse or repeated episodes with such a loss of control are signals of serious problems in an individual, relationship, or marriage and will destroy the trust that is required of a healthy sexual relationship. Emotional abuse will eventually erode a person's feelings of love and sexual desire for their partner. In this case, the problem is usually not simply a difference in sexual desire, but a problem with the relationship or marriage.

If you have found yourselves in a cycle of sexual power struggles, you are not alone and your situation is not hopeless! The Ten Minute Sexual Solution is about helping you as a couple to break free from your sexual power struggles and find new, innovative, and successful ways to deal with your differences in sexual desire. For the lower-desire partner, in most cases, know this: You are not sexually dead! While it might be true that you do have a lower sexual desire than your partner, and that after months (or years) of sexual badgering, your desire changed from low to nonexistent, you can still revive your dormant sexual self, like a phoenix that rises from the ashes.

The truth may be that you don't actually have a problem with low sexual desire. You may have lower sexual desire or different sexual desires than your partner, but you may still be "normal." The truth may be that you experience sexual desire differently than other people, which will be explained in chapter 8. If you have been the one coerced into having unwanted sex and you no longer enjoy sex, take heart, and be patient. You are probably not sexually dead; your sexual self is simply lost. You can find your sexual self again, or find it for the first time. The good news is that low sexual desire can often be changed!

SEXUAL SOLUTIONS TO SEXUAL POWER STRUGGLES

The cycle of a sexual power struggle must first be broken in order to avoid painful emotional and sexual consequences in your relationship. Many people get stuck in emotional fears and irrational assumptions as the lower-/higher-desire partner. The solution is to find the real reasons behind low sexual desire and solve them, or manage differences in sexual desires to have a healthy sexual relationship.

Each partner needs to create his/her own sexual identity as unique as his/her own personality, with his/her own needs, desires and wants, and learn to accept, understand, and work together as a team for sexual change in the relationship. Every couple will have sexual differences over the course of a long-term relationship or marriage. Every couple needs to learn sexual communication to share their sexual selves with each other. The Ten Minute Sexual Solution starts with first learning to talk about sex, then making a commitment to work on new sexual solutions that do not include sexual coercion, badgering, or sexual passive-aggressiveness. You can stop taking desperate measures to change your sex life by learning to directly communicate and negotiate with each other in a loving way to share a more intimate and passionate relationship.

As you read through the book, you will find many solutions to create sexual desire, deal with differences in sexual desire, and increase your sexual pleasure and frequency. Chapter 7 introduces maintenance sex, which helps couples who have sexual differences or are out of sync to develop sexual synchronicity. More information on the emotional consequences of sexual power struggles is found in chapters 9 and 10, addressing men and women (and higher-/lower-desire partners) individually. For now, seek to find the causes of and solutions for the real problem: different or low sexual desire.

PART II: CAUSES AND TYPES OF LOW SEXUAL DESIRE

If you have a low sex or sexless relationship, the chances are very good that one of you has low sexual desire, the most common cause of low sexual frequency. If you are going to fix your sexless relationship, you need to find out if one of you is having a problem with low sexual desire and why. Since low sexual desire or inhibited sexual desire (ISD) is a common sexual problem, affecting 15 percent of men[1] and 33 percent of women[2] and their sexual partners, it will be helpful to have a better understanding of an individual's problem. Since sexual desire can be affected by a couple's relationship, the end of this section summarizes these factors.

First, you need to figure out exactly what is causing your problem with low sexual desire. If you're not having sex very often or not at all, you might already know that one of you has a problem with low sexual desire. But before you move on to figuring out how to solve the problem, **you need to be sure you are working on the right problem**. I *strongly recommend* that you first make sure your problem is actually, specifically, about sexual desire, or you may be wasting your time and energy and get frustrated over your lack of success in changing your sex life. You can work all day on fine tuning and turbo-charging the engine of your car to give it power, but if the car is missing a major part, such as a battery or steering wheel, then you can't drive it. The same is true with sexual desire: Make sure you're working on the right problem to get the right results.

TEN MINUTE TIP

Although many reasons for low sexual desire are presented, pay attention to the very important section "One Simple Explanation to Sexual Pain." Sexual pain inhibits sexual desire. In my practice, the most common cause of pain for women is not a complex medical problem; it is because they are not physically ready for sexual intercourse. Many people do not understand some basic facts about how a woman's body works during sex, which, when learned, often easily resolves the problem!

Usually, the diagnosis of low sexual desire is easily identified, but the cause is more difficult to determine. Sometimes the causes are not known consciously, and there are often multiple and complex reasons for low sexual desire. The complexity of sexual desire is sometimes as diverse as each person's personality, and in fact, it is often a reflection of the individual's personality. In this section, we'll look at the major factors that contribute to low sexual desire, ruling out other sexual dysfunctions that cause low sexual desire (or might be your real problem). The Ten Minute Sexual Solution will work far better for you if you address any barriers or problems that need to be solved first.

What Exactly IS Low Sexual Desire?

Let's start with the medical definition, adapted from the Diagnostic Statistical Manual for Mental Disorders, DSM-IV-TR[3]:

Hypoactive Sexual Desire Disorder

- Desire for and fantasies about sexual activity are chronically or recurrently diminished or absent, and:
- This behavior causes marked distress or interpersonal problems.
- Except for another Sexual Dysfunction, no other mental health disorder, such as depression or anxiety or personality problems, explains it better.
- It is not directly caused by substance use (medication or drug or alcohol abuse) or by a general medical condition.

Classifications of Low Sexual Desire

- Primary low sexual desire: You have always had no or low sexual desire.
- Secondary low sexual desire: You once had sexual desire, but you no longer have sexual desire.
- Situational low sexual desire: In some situations you feel desire, while in others, you don't. A common example, is some women feel sexual desire and choose to masturbate regularly, but have no desire for sex with their partners. Another example is when a person has no desire for sex with his or her partner, but seeks extramarital affairs and feels a great deal of sexual desire.

First, you have to rule out that your low sexual desire is not the result of a medical condition, such as low sexual arousal or sexual pain, or due to psychiatric problems, such as depression or personality disorders. Obviously, if your desire for sex is simply not there or has dramatically decreased, you do have a problem with low sexual desire. However, you want to make sure that you understand the primary cause in order to increase the chances that specific treatment for low sexual desire will work for you. Resolving the primary problem may spontaneously solve the low sexual desire, or you may need to work on that separately after solving other problems. Most people have to work on solving the problem of low sexual desire while working with other problems. For example, in the case of depression, one works on medically treating depression while working on enhancing your sexual relationship. First, rule out other explanations for low sexual desire before beginning to work on your relationship or practicing the tips in this book for creating sexual desire.

SEXUAL PROBLEMS THAT CAUSE OR EXPLAIN LOW SEXUAL DESIRE

SEXUAL PAIN

Frequently, when women have a problem with low sexual desire, one finds a problem of having pain with sexual intercourse. Let's be real! If something hurts…you don't want it!

> **Sexual pain for women is REAL and needs to be addressed FIRST, when it comes to your sexual relationship.**

Sexual pain is different than low sexual desire, but when sex hurts, you either want to avoid sex or you don't desire it. When a woman says that sex hurts, the sexual desire problem may be due to pain and usually is not due to an inherent problem with sexual desire or wanting her partner. Amazingly, many couples have never discussed the problem of sexual pain or discomfort, or realized that is why an individual doesn't want or avoids sex. Often, a woman is secretly in pain, not telling her partner, and her partner has no idea that it is a serious problem. Sometimes the woman feels embarrassed or inadequate, thinking that she should like sex, so she just doesn't talk about it. Sometimes a woman wants to please her partner and wants to give sexual pleasure, so she doesn't speak up when she begins to feel pain. She might think sex won't last that much longer, that she can handle a little bit of discomfort, but it turns out to hurt more than she thought it would. In the long run, she will remember the pain and avoid more frequent sex.

TWO MAJOR CATEGORIES OF SEXUAL PAIN

- Dyspareunia. A woman often experiences genital pain with sexual intercourse, but such pain is attributable neither to vaginismus (see below) nor to inadequate lubrication. One example is vulvadynia, which is vulvular pain.
- Vaginismus. The woman repeatedly has spasms of the vaginal muscles that interfere with sexual intercourse. Basically, a woman's pelvic floor muscles "clamp down" and hurt, and vaginal penetration is impossible or very painful. Women with vaginismus often have difficulty having sexual intercourse. Vaginismus is beyond the scope of this book, but you can find more information about it in *Sex Matters for Women*[4].

Sexual pain can be complex and difficult to resolve. The very first step to solving a sexual pain problem is to stop having sexual intercourse or sexual activity that is painful. In almost all sex therapy cases, a woman with sexual pain is referred for medical attention with her gynecologist and help from a professionally trained sex therapist.

ONE SIMPLE EXPLANATION FOR SEXUAL PAIN

In many cases in my sex therapy practice, women who have been referred for treatment of sexual pain do not have a complex medical condition or sexual dysfunction. In fact, many women who ask to be treated for low sexual desire have been found to have sexual pain that can be easily resolved. In many cases, sexual pain has been found to be caused by the fact that the woman is not physically excited or ready for sex! Many people do not know about how a woman's body responds to sex when she is not sexually excited, (lubricated or "wet" and aroused), but it is a very common reason for sexual discomfort and pain. I cannot emphasize how important this information and section is to understanding low sexual desire and sexual frequency. A vast majority of women with low sexual desire due to sexual pain can be easily "treated," when they learn the truth about the cause of their sexual pain!

ONE ESSENTIAL SEXUAL SOLUTION FOR SEXUAL PAIN

The Problem: When a woman becomes sexually aroused, that is, sexually excited, her vagina lubricates or "gets wet," her vaginal tissue becomes engorged with blood making it softer and more pliable, and her vagina expands about two inches longer. The average woman's vagina is four inches deep. Sexually excited, her vagina is, on average, six inches deep. The average man's penis, erect, is six inches long. If the average woman is sexually aroused and excited, she will normally be able to feel comfortable accommodating the average man's erection for sexual intercourse. If the woman is not excited, sexual penetration with intercourse will include the man's six-inch erection thrusting deep inside a four-inch pocket of dry, tight skin, and quickly hitting against the back of her vagina onto her hard cervix, which can be felt by all of the surrounding organs, including the uterus, bladder, and even vibrationally up to her tonsils and down to her toes. This causes sexual pain that is real, and it hurts. A woman needs to be sexually excited and physically aroused in order to have lubrication and expansion of her vagina, prior to having sexual intercourse.

Many women experience pain during intercourse for years before they finally shut down physically and emotionally and decide that they have low/no sexual desire. Also, when a woman is not sexually aroused and her vagina has not expanded, simply using a lubricant to prepare for sexual intercourse will not be enough for comfortable sex. Lubricants will not make the vagina expand. Having intercourse while the woman is not actually physically aroused will still result in the man's penis hitting the back of the vagina or cervix, pounding against her body, which causes sexual discomfort and pain.

With this type of sexual pain problem, the real problem is a lack of sexual arousal or excitement or an inability to get excited. In most cases, the cause is a lack of adequate sexual foreplay, an inability to get aroused, a lack of personal knowledge about how to get sexual excited, or an emotional or mental resistance resulting from difficulties in your relationship.

The Solution: First, if you are having sexual pain, try to have more foreplay, initially spending at least 20 minutes on foreplay before you try to have sexual penetration or intercourse. Start with non-sexual touching, such as kissing and caressing, then progress to direct sexual stimulation, such as manual stimulation of the genitals and oral sex. Non-sexual touching exercises are further discussed in chapter 5. If you are personally not able to get aroused, go to chapter 8 to learn how to have sexual pleasure, arousal, and orgasms. If none of these suggestions help, you might address issues in your relationship that may be leading you to anger or anxiety with your partner, which can inhibit sexual arousal.

If you are having pain with intercourse that is not explained by the description above, you may be having physical pain that needs to be addressed by your gynecologist. If you have never been sexually aroused, despite repeated experiences with sexual stimulation, you might have a problem with sexual arousal, and you will want to consult a sex therapist and/or gynecologist. Sexual pain may also come from endometriosis, vaginismus, sexually transmitted infections, or urethra infections, for example.

TEN MINUTE TIP

If you are having sexual pain, consult your gynecologist. Try to have your gynecologist replicate that pain in the office, so you can determine the location of your sexual pain. During your gynecological examination, allow your doctor to try to penetrate or gently press against the walls just outside or just inside your vagina, and see if you feel the same kind of pain that you have during sexual intercourse. You need to let your doctor know if and/or when you feel physical discomfort and report that pain to your doctor. Sometimes this pain can be replicated, and sometimes it cannot be replicated, even when it is present. Using this information, your doctor may be able to help you pinpoint the cause of your pain. If your doctor tells you that "there is nothing wrong with you," and you know you are having sexual pain, I strongly recommend that you seek the professional help of a sex therapist (aasect.org). In addition, there are sexual pain clinics that specialize in working with women.

LOW SEXUAL AROUSAL OR EXCITEMENT

Both men and women can experience low sexual arousal. Low sexual arousal is when one does not get sexually excited and/or does not respond to sexual touch or stimulation. For men, sexual excitement it defined as being able to have or maintain an erection sufficient to engage in intercourse. For women, low sexual arousal is clinically defined as an inability to become vaginally lubricated, but it generally means that one does not get "turned on." Contrary to popular belief, a lack of lubrication is not always caused by a failure to be aroused. A woman may feel sexually excited but not have lubrication. The exact causes of female sexual arousal disorder are unknown.

Arousal disorders have been associated with illness, a lack of the hormones estrogen and testosterone, and side effects from medications. Possible psychological explanations include sexual guilt, hostility, anxiety, and relationship problems. For both men and women, problems with sexual arousal can be confused with sexual desire, but there might not be a sexual desire problem at all. When people are not able to respond to sexual touch, get excited, or have orgasms, they might not be interested in sex and feel no sexual desire. On the other hand, if they enjoyed sex, they might actually begin to want and desire sex, which is often the case in my practice. Arousal disorders often require professional help from a sex therapist and/or a gynecologist.

SEXUAL AVERSION

Sexual aversion is very different than low sexual desire. It is a sexual dysfunction in which, to an extreme degree, one dislikes and avoids nearly all genital contact with a sex partner. Specifically, a person feels very averse to, repulsed by, or hates sex itself. In fact, with sexual aversion there is often a physical reaction against sex, including feeling nauseas, wanting to react with anger physically (such as feeling like hitting someone if they get close to them sexually) or literally wanting to run away or hide from sexual situations.

Sexual aversion is often associated with a history of sexual abuse or trauma, but not always. Low sexual desire and sexual aversion are two distinctly different types of sexual problems, and are treated differently as well. While sexual aversion may be situational, such as when a person is averse to a spouse who has raped her, it is more often generalized and associated with any person or partner. It is highly recommended that a person with sexual aversion seek professional treatment with a certified sex therapist.

MEDICAL CAUSES FOR SEXUAL DESIRE AND AROUSAL PROBLEMS

You have to rule out medical causes for your sexual problem before you take on the Ten Minute Sexual Solution. If you have any medical problems or are taking any medications, consult your physician and ask how your medical condition or medication might affect sexuality. Common medical problems include depression, menopause, prostate cancer or infections, hypothyroidism, panic disorders, bipolar disorders, stroke, alcoholism, and other addictions. Consult your pharmacist, read the lengthy inserts of drug information, or consult the Internet regarding your specific medication. The following drug categories are known to decrease sexual desire: Blood pressure medications, cancer drugs, tranquilizers such as Xanax, anti-depressants, and chronic use of recreational drugs such as alcohol and cocaine. If you are taking any medications, find out if they are decreasing your sexual desire. In most cases, get a full medical check up and rule out physical causes for sexual desire and sexual excitement problems.

You can see that your problem may truly be that one or both of you has low sexual desire, but it may be that you have a completely different sexual problem or dysfunction altogether. After you have ruled out, or treated these medical problems, then move on to find out how to work on rekindling sexual desire in your relationship.

COUPLES AND LOW SEXUAL DESIRE

The truth is, many clients I see are fine sexually—that is, they were until they got married or into a committed long-term relationship and their sex drives changed. It's a chicken and the egg story: What came first? Was it the lack of sexual desire or the relationship conflicts that killed your sex life? Most clients that I see with low sexual desire have one or more of the following problems.

- Relationship problems that suppress (or kill) their sexual desire. Betrayals (cheating or addictions), no emotional intimacy, disagreements/resentments over household chores, kids, money, in-laws, communication, and the fighting/sexual power struggles that follows these problems cause desire problems. Chapters 4 to 7 will help you address many of these problems, but some couples may need to seek therapy, especially when dealing with sexual infidelity.

- One person has a problem with no or slow arousal and/or orgasms or sexual pain that suppresses desire because there's little sexual pleasure. Resolving medical problems first, then working on creating sexual desire (in chapters 8 to 10) helps with this problem.
- Individual psychological barriers to wanting/loving sex. For example: a strict religious background that created sexual guilt, distrust from past relationships, or past sexual trauma. Sex therapy is recommended.
- Attraction: A couple was never attracted to each other or lost their attraction.

All of the other factors above are covered in this chapter or book, or are beyond the scope of this book (e.g. psychological and sexual trauma, affairs), except for the matter of attraction. Attraction is a difficult but essential topic to address in the cause of low sexual desire, before beginning the Ten Minute Sexual Solution.

ATTRACTION

In the very first sex therapy session, I almost always try to find out if my clients are really attracted to their sexual partners or spouses. When couples come to therapy with the problem of low sexual frequency or desire, it is important to find out if they love each other or if they were ever in love or ever really attracted to each other. If you know you are attracted to each other, skip to the next section. Although it is not a common factor among the complex reasons for low sexual desire, despite it quite commonly being a fear with couples, attraction is an important component of sexual desire. At times, I am surprised by the many reasons that couples get together that have nothing to do with being attracted to each other. Generally, if you were once attracted to your partner, but your feelings have changed, you may very well be able to rekindle that attraction; but if you were never attracted, or you're not really that attracted to your partner, you are not likely to develop sexual desire for them.

- Were you ever really attracted to your partner?
- Are you currently attracted to your partner?
- Were/are you really passionate or hot for your partner?

Attraction is loosely defined here as physical attraction, but it is also emotional attraction; however, it is not like what you feel toward your brother or sister or roommate.

THE CIRCLE OF ATTRACTION

Think of a "circle of attraction" like a dart board with a bulls–eye in the middle and a series of outside circles surrounding it. The bulls–eye is your ideal of physical, emotional, and sexual attraction. Each of the outside circles has a decreasing value, like points on a dart board. Somebody is going to fit your "center of attraction," or bulls–eye. For some people, it's Johnny Depp or Ellen DeGeneres or Paris Hilton. Now, I don't expect that you are going to be dating movie stars, but you need to know what you like (or don't like).

TEN MINUTE TIP

Draw a dartboard and place an "X" on the spot for your partner, for how close they were to the bulls-eye, at the height of your attraction to them. For some people, their partner falls right in the center, in the bulls-eye. This is someone you feel very attracted to, you feel very comfortable, with or they "complete you." If this is your situation, you are very lucky. If your X is close to the center, then you are like most people in relationships. If you are a few circles off, you might be in trouble, because here is the secret: Your original feelings of attraction are a constant. The distance between the bulls-eye and your X is likely to remain the same over time.

Your original feelings don't change a great deal. Oh, your feelings can change and diminish depending on the situation or over time, when you're mad at someone, feel betrayed, or you've drifted apart. The good news is, if you once had strong feelings of attraction for someone, you can get back to where you once were at your best of times by working on the steps of the Ten Minute Sexual Solution. But if your X is way off center, and was from the very beginning, and you were never attracted to your partner there is nothing that any person, or sex therapist, can do to make you feel attracted to your partner.

So ask yourself, "Was I ever sexually attracted to my current partner?" If the answer is no, then you probably have a serious problem that will limit and affect your sexual desire for your partner. For some reason, you settled down or possibly married someone that you were not that "hot for" or not "totally into," that was never close to your center of attraction. Examples include people who married for safety or security, because of an unplanned pregnancy, good timing, or to save themselves from homosexuality. Conversely, if you've drifted off from where you once were at best, you can get back to or close to where you began by working on the steps in *The Ten Minute Sexual Solution* to renew, rekindle, and recreate your intimacy and passion.

CHAPTER

3

A Guide to *The Ten Minute Sexual Solution*

Sexual silence about emotionally and sexually distant relation-ships creates a secret shame. No one wants to admit membership in the nameless, faceless club of couples who have somehow lost their sexual passion. Sexual secrets are the best kept in the world. The answer to shame is a powerful truth: Sexual solutions are real and some are very simple. Many people can change their intimate relationships and sexual lives with innovative sexual solutions that you can use in just ten minutes a day starting now!

My husband and I are both couples and sex therapists, but we are also real people. We have five children between us, three that live with us, sometimes four, plus the kids' friends, three jobs, two yards, three parents, ten brothers and sisters, twenty-eight nieces and nephews, birthdays, holidays, traveling sports teams, a house and a very old, small office building to maintain. Our clients think that since we're both sex therapists, we must be having sex all the time! However, since we don't get home from work until 8 P.M. some nights, or we have been working all day, then picking up someone from practice, going home to fix dinner, then starting on homework (often for hours with two A.D.D. children), while doing the laundry between math problems, we tend to be a little on the tired side during the week. Or plain old totally exhausted. Just like our clients, and just like you: We are real, busy people.

Necessity is the mother of invention. We invented the Ten Minute Sexual Solution to figure out how to stay connected as a couple, keep our love alive, and maintain a happy, healthy, frequent sex life. We needed an economy of emotional intimacy and sex powerful enough to sustain a great love, simple enough for an ADD spouse to remember, and brief enough to fit into real life responsibilities, without losing the benefits of true love and passionate sex.

As marriage and sex therapists, we found many busy couples with the same time and energy problems in their relationships as we experienced. Over time, many couples have found the Ten Minute Sexual Solution has helped them get their friendship back, improve intimacy, put their sex life back on track, find sexual synchronicity, saved their marriage or relationship, and helped them enjoy a life-long commitment to sexuality and intimacy. Almost everyone can use some of these techniques to manage the stressful, busy aspects of real life for real couples.

WHAT IS THE TEN MINUTE SEXUAL SOLUTION?

This chapter provides an overview to the Ten Minute Sexual Solution, including the process of creating a foundation of intimacy to pave the path for passionate lovemaking and maintenance sex. Subsequent chapters will provide the detailed information and 10 minute solutions you need to build your skills and knowledge and create intimacy and passion in your relationship.

The Ten Minute Sexual Solution is a five-step process to change your relationship and set a foundation for sexual change for real couples. In 10 minutes a day, you can learn and practice sexual communication skills, deepen emotional intimacy, stop and resolve conflicts, and learn new approaches to creating sexual desire, all to improve your relationship and increase your sexual frequency. At the end of this chapter, a one month program outlines specific "sexercises" to complete on a week to week basis, to give you a guide to creating intimacy and passion as a busy couple.

FIVE STEPS TO THE TEN MINUTE SEXUAL SOLUTION

1. **Learn the secrets of sexual communication.** Develop your sexual voice, and then practice sexual communication as a couple. Men and women *both* need to develop a sexual voice and say what they really want and what they don't want. To really take care of each other, you need to know where each other is at sexually, and to what degree are you sexually frustrated or in need of intimacy and closeness. So learn to let each other know exactly where you stand, sexually speaking. The program starts with chapter 4 where you will learn 10 minute solutions for sexual communication.

2. **Creating a solid foundation of intimacy.** Make your relationship work outside the bedroom first. Work on the other intimacy aspects of a relationship besides sex to increase your desire for sexual intimacy. Take Dr. Darcy's "Intimacy Test" and rate your relationship before and after you begin working on your relationship, when you get to chapter 5. Practice sexercises to learn several 10 minute solutions for creating couple closeness!

3. **Learn to fight right.** Anger is the number one killer of sexual desire. Learn to fight fair and resolve a conflict when you disagree. If you have a problem with having too many arguments, it can ruin your intimacy and relationship and kill your sexual relationship. Leftover anger and resentments lead to less affection, a lack of touching, and a decreased desire to make love. Chapter 6 teaches you 10

essential steps on how to fight right. Don't push anger under the rug: It usually ends up under the covers.

4. **Create sexual desire.** Together and individually, work on understanding and creating sexual desire for yourself and your partner. The solutions can range from amazingly simple to very complex. Start with chapter 2 to understand the effect of sexual power struggles on low sexual desire in some couple's relationships. Chapter 2 provides very important information on the different causes and types of low sexual desire that need to be identified, as well as some solutions to resolve sexual barriers for individuals and couples. Chapter 8 introduces innovative approaches to creating sexual desire. Chapters 9 and 10 teach lower-desire partners how to awaken their sexual selves and show both couples and individuals how to understand and change higher-desire relationship dynamics.

5. **Maintenance sex for busy couples.** Maintenance sex can be a part of your new, loving sexual relationship, and a bridge to resolve your sexual differences. Imagine sexual synchronicity. You can learn a new way to approach and please each other, in light of your different sexual drives. Maintenance sex can be a less threatening way to really make your relationship work sexually. You can discover how to share sexual accommodation and become sexually different partners with each other. After creating a foundation of sexual communication and emotional intimacy, learn about maintenance sex for busy couples in chapter 7.

SPECIAL CONDITIONS FOR PARENTS: BEYOND THE TEN MINUTE SEXUAL SOLUTION

Couples with children have more difficulty finding 10 minutes in their day to find their way to sexual play! Here are some special conditions for the Ten Minute Sexual Solution to make it work for you. You're a real couple with busy lives and yet real needs to be just a woman, a man, and a couple, too. The 10 minute sexercises found in *The Ten Minute Sexual Solution* are designed with you in mind—to have time for yourself, your relationship and, really, for your children, too!

The greatest gift that you can give your children is to be happy!

Your children's happiness includes your being happy, showing them how to be happy, and keeping your family together. Being happy in your relationship or marriage is great for your life, and great for your children's lives, too. You are teaching your child how to have a relationship in the future by how you relate to each other as parents now. You are teaching them about love. Make love a priority in your life. Do not be hesitant to have "adult time," making it as high a priority as your kids' homework time, basketball or dance practice, dinner time, or story time. You certainly spend more than 10 minutes a day in all of these activities. Let your children know that your relationship or marriage is just as important as their time with friends and playtime. Have adult playtime and don't feel guilty about it! You are teaching them about adult-sized love!

Have an "Adult-Centered" family instead of a "Child-Centered" family—at least sometimes!

1. **Adult time.** Make time-outs for "adult time." This means adult-only conversations without interruptions, dates and dinner out without the kids, uninterrupted phone calls, and bath time. Whatever your meaning of "adult time," let it be known that adults want their own time to

be people, separate from being parents, even for 10 minutes at a time!

2. **Privacy.** Put a lock on your bedroom door and use it. So many couples either do not have a lock or they are reluctant to use it. They do not want their door locked when their child comes to the door after bedtime to ask for a glass of water or a second hug. Many people think it gives the kids the wrong idea. Wrong. First of all, with our five children, and lots of teaching and reminders, we have found that kids "forget" to knock and walk, run, or fall into our room without blinking an eye. It really is okay to let kids know that sometimes you want privacy, perhaps because you are dressing or just want alone time for yourself and as a couple. It is a good message to give to your children that there is a boundary between parents and children at times, even if for only 10 minutes. When your children are teenagers, they will lock their doors sometimes, too, just to feel like an independent person for a few minutes. You can unlock the door at night, when you are ready to sleep, for safety reasons.

3. **Bedtime**. Put the children to bed on time. Children need a bedtime, for themselves and for you. Make it at least one hour before you go to bed, if not sooner. Adults need time to wind down, and children need more time to sleep than adults. If the kids go to bed at 8:30 and you go to bed at 10:00, you have 90 minutes to spend time together as adults. You do not always need to sort socks at 10 P.M. Give yourselves a break as parents and do NOT always watch TV, spend time on the computer, or do chores after the kids go to bed. Look at each other, talk to each other, and, well, go to bed, even if one person gets back up and stays up later than the other because of different schedules or sleep habits.

3. **The noise-buster.** Put a CD player or TV in your bedroom to cut down on "noise" that will make you self-conscious when you have children within potential earshot. Use the electronics randomly, so the kids don't think you only listen to music when mom and dad are alone. When your tots turn in to teens, you don't want them to turn into the "sex police," who come knocking on your door late at night. Give them

a noise-buster, such as a radio or wireless headphones to wear late at night, when they "can't sleep."

4. **The Sex Police.** What are you going to do about the Sex Police? I'm talking about your kids…when they find out you have sex! What do you do when your kids hear you making noises in your bedroom and they knock on your door, or they walk in on the "primal scene," or they mention something as a "joke" in passing about you and sex? Suddenly, you realize that your kids know you are a sexual person! If this happens, you will need to have a talk with your kids. You may want to buy a book on sexuality that is appropriate for your kids, such as *It's Perfectly Normal,*[1] by Robie Harris (ages 10 and up) or *Virgin Sex for Girls*[2]*/Guys*[3] (ages 13-20) by Dr. Darcy Luadzers.

Depending on your child's age and maturity, be honest with them about sexuality, and focus on respecting each other's privacy. Remember, no matter how normal and healthy sex is, when it comes to sex and parents there is just a definite cultural "gross-out" factor. Whether you have little kids shoving their toy cars under your locked door, wondering when you are going to come out and play, or you have teenagers who make some kind of mocking "sex noise" (like banging on the walls as a joke and rolling their eyes upwards, whether you had sex or not!) when you come out of your bedroom, you have to deal with the sex police!

TAKING ON THE TEN MINUTE SEXUAL SOLUTION

CHARLIE AND ELIZA'S STORY

Charlie was 48 years old and his bride of three years was 46. Charlie moved out and into a hotel after telling Eliza, "I'm not living in another sexless marriage." Charlie had been married to his first wife for 20 years. The last 10 years of their marriage, they never had sex more than once or twice a year, but he felt he had to stay married to raise their children. Eliza had been single for many years, after her first brief marriage to a man who turned out to prefer men over women. She knew what it was like to live with someone who didn't want her and to feel sexually rejected. When Charlie and Eliza dated, they had sex all the time. In fact, Eliza was often the initiator and was sexually aggressive. Charlie could hardly keep up with her, to the point that he said, "Well, I've met my match!" Beside sex, the two had a lot in common, working in a similar profession for many years.

The separation was devastating to Eliza, who had been madly in love with Charlie when they married three years earlier. When they were dating they had great sex, often several times a week. But on the honeymoon, the first hint of trouble started. They had had sex on their wedding night and the following day. On the third next day, Charlie asked to have sex again. Eliza answered, "Do we have to have sex EVERY day?" Charlie was shocked at the rejection, got mad and said, for the first time in their marriage, "I'm not asking for sex every day, but I'm not having another sexless marriage, either!" That moment was filled with a great deal of tension, anxiety, and prophecy for the next few years of their marriage.

After the honeymoon, "normal life" seemed to set in: dealing with work, their children from their previous marriages, and day to day life. In addition, Eliza started going through menopause, and she completely lost interest in sex. Their sex life dwindled down to one or two times a month, in a good month.

Charlie loved Eliza and wanted to be with her, but he was not willing to live in a marriage without a "normal sexual relationship," which he thought meant having sex a few times a week. Eliza loved Charlie, but she could not stand his sexual demands and felt so much sexual pressure from him that she didn't ever feel like having sex anymore. Eliza felt like their entire relationship revolved around sex, rather than all the great things they seemed to have in common when they were dating. Eliza also felt guilty because she was going through hormonal changes and she just couldn't seem to "make herself want sex."

Eliza and Charlie came in for sex therapy. Beside low sexual frequency, their relationship was strained from the fights over sex. In addition, for Charlie, sex was equated with love. He felt that if his wife really loved him, then she would want to have sex with him frequently, at least a few times a week. Plus, Charlie simply didn't want a sexless marriage. Eliza wanted to want sex, but she had low sexual desire hormonally and any other sexual desire was squashed by sexual pressure she felt from Charlie, which currently meant "put out or I'll divorce you." Eliza felt resentful towards Charlie for "blackmailing her for sex," especially when she was having a medical problem with sexual desire.

Eliza and Charlie really were attracted to each other, loved each other, had a lot in common, and wanted to have a life together. Eliza had only a brief first marriage, and then she had a single life for 20 years, having brief and longer affairs and intense sexual relationships, but no long-term relationships. Charlie had only known one long marriage, and one brief and intense sexual affair that lasted several months before he met Eliza. Both Eliza and Charlie needed to learn how to manage a sexual relationship in a long-term relationship, which is completely different than dating. Married sex involves intense, passionate sex, but it also includes married sex and maintenance sex. Maintenance sex requires sexual communication and agreements about sexually accommodating your partner, even when one partner is not that interested or thinking about sex at the time.

Charlie and Eliza first had to learn to communicate about sexual needs. Charlie had shut down, gotten resentful and angry, and had periodic angry outbursts toward Eliza. In turn, this made Eliza shut down sexually even more, feeling intimidated by Charlie. She felt like she had to have sex with him or he'd get angry, and then there would be a nasty scene. Neither Charlie nor Eliza had very much experience with saying what they really wanted sexually, how much they wanted or didn't want it, on a daily basis. Fortunately, both of them were good communicators, and with practice they learned how to communicate their thoughts and feelings about sex, as well as other minor matters in their marriage.

Because of the unresolved sexual conflicts, Charlie and Eliza began avoiding each other in their marriage, spent their nights in different parts of their house, and they shared very little affection, touching, or even time together. In the beginning of therapy, regaining their intimate relationship, without the pressure of sex, was important to rekindle their loving feelings for each other. Overcoming the emotional distance and resolving their resentments took several weeks to accomplish. Using the Ten Minute Sexual Solution, Charlie and Eliza focused on spending at least 10 minutes a day on caring behaviors toward each other, to foster their affection and intimacy.

After a month, because Eliza's lower sexual desire interfered with a "normal" sex drive, they agreed to share maintenance sex at least once a week to accommodate Charlie's sexual needs, even if Eliza really wasn't in the mood for sex. By sharing maintenance sex, they more than doubled their sexual frequency in only a matter of weeks. Sometimes Eliza really enjoyed sex, and other times it was just about being Charlie's lover, being there for him, and feeling close to him, even for just 10 minutes. At less frequent times, once a month or so,

Eliza did have sexual desire, got into sex, and they had a fireworks session of sex that lasted longer and made Charlie feel wanted. Maintenance sex helped Charlie and Eliza bridge their sexual gap and create greater sexual synchronicity. They resolved many of their conflicts and anger, which helped them deal with menopause, too. The Ten Minute Sexual Solution helped them to share the love the felt for each other, without robbing them of their marriage.

A ONE MONTH PROGRAM TO CREATE INTIMACY AND PASSION

Sex therapy is not a secret science. The great news is that the Ten Minute Sexual Solution is a sex therapy program that almost anyone can use to improve their relationship and sexual relationship. What would take you years to learn in a classroom or months in couples and sex therapy is condensed into easy-to-learn steps to relationship and sexual healing. This program launches new approaches to sex therapy for couples, including creating sexual desire and creating sexual synchronicity through maintenance sex. The topics and homework assignments are brought to you straight from the couch of a real sex therapist. All of the "sexercises" have been used in the course of couples and sex therapy for thousands of people, exploring and working on the same problems you experience in your relationship.

> **You can be your own sex therapist!**

In sex therapy, you would get a more individualized plan, depending on your personalities, the goals of therapy, and your needs and pace of progress as a couple. Since that isn't possible here, you will get to experience many different types of communication, intimacy, and sexual exercises used to help couples regain emotional intimacy and a sexual relationship. Some of them will work incredibly well for you, while others may not be needed by you personally. Sex therapists have their own therapy styles and treatment interventions that will often vary on many of these same themes. Working with a certified sex therapist can save you time and give you emotional support to solve problem areas that you can't easily see on your own, so some readers may choose to follow up with one of the many gifted and sensitive sex therapists or counselors (look at aasect.org for one in your area). However, many people don't have a local neighborhood sex therapist, or they can't afford to pay hundreds or thousands of dollars to see one. With this program, you can work at being your own sex therapists. You may be amazed at your progress, working together in the context of your personal relationship from the privacy of your own home.

WORKING THE PROGRAM

First, start by reading the book. It's a novel concept, but you will want to understand the whole picture before you get started. Read the book all the way through, then come back to working the program. If your partner chooses to read the book with you, GREAT! Ideally, you will each read the book, or you can even read it together. If not, you can work on the sexercises together anyway. *The Ten Minute Sexual Solution* is designed to help couples jump start their intimacy and sexual relationship by devoting 10 minutes a day to changing your sex life. This program outlines the sexercises for couples to complete together week to week. The sexercises are found with detailed explanations in chapters 4 through 10. The exercises build on one another, so learning one skill is important to master before you try the next one.

"S-EXERCISES"

If you are like my clients, you are probably thinking, "Yeah, that sounds great, but what do I DO?" You will be given very specific step-by-step directions, called, since this *is* a sex therapy program, "sexercises," showing you what you can do and what you can try, to find what works for you. Some couples will be able to follow the program, down to the day-to-day details, to make real changes in their relationship. Some couples may use the program as a guide to make changes over a longer period of time, while other couples will only need to take on a few of the tasks before they find their relationship changing in a positive way. You can work the program systematically or not, but in order to be successful, it is very important that you complete the sexercises on developing communication and intimacy first, prior to starting on any sexual exercises.

SEXERCISES GUIDELINES:

- You can double up and complete two or three of the assignments at one time, or simply take them one day at a time, depending on how you schedule your time.
- Do take turns initiating sexercises, unless the sexercise directly tells you who is responsible for getting things started. It is strongly recommended that you decide in advance who will initate each of the sexercises.
- Some couples like to take an hour and work on a few things at once, then wait another week or until the weekend to move on to the next homework exercise. Take it at your pace, but don't try to do too many things in one day.
- Do try to do at least one sexercise twice a week!
- Do set deadlines for completing homework, such as completing all the "weekly" exercises in one week or even two weeks. Deadlines can remind couples to complete their sexercises on a regular basis, even if you turn this into a two month program. Often, in sex therapy, couples finish their homework the night before a session (their deadline), just like homework in high school or college. Try to avoid this.
- Let your relationship change over time, rather than trying to force change suddenly, and it will seem like a more natural way to have

fun together instead of work. Many couples are seen every other week, allowing change to occur more gradually, creating a two month program.

- Additional sexercises are found in the last two chapters that target more specific problem areas and are not a part of the one month program. These can be completed over time or as needed to progress toward your individual goals.

IMPORTANT GUIDELINE: TAKE A SEXUAL BREAK! With most couples, I recommend that they discontinue having sexual relations for the first month, including any sexual touch that is not a part of a sexercise. Agreeing to delay sex until after you finish all of the sexercises in the one month program is often essential, if not helpful, to relieve sexual pressure and tension in your relationship and develop sexual trust. Delaying sex will allow you to be more successful in experiencing more emotional closeness, as well as feeling safety and trust to share non-sexual physical affection. For couples with sexless relationships delaying sex is usually not a big problem, since you aren't having sex more than once a month anyway. Many lower-desire partners are afraid to ask for this sexual break, but almost always higher-desire partners are very understanding and accommodating. You may agree that either of you may choose to masturbate alone during this time. Although it might sound like you are going backwards in order to go forwards, I highly recommend you follow the guideline, especially if one of the partners has a low sexual desire.

THE TEN MINUTE SEXUAL SOLUTION

WEEK ONE: Sexual Communication
(All sexercises in chapter 4)
Day 1–2: Sexercise #1: The Sex Talk
Day 2: Sexercise #2: Sexual Language
Day 3: Sexercise #3: Making a Commitment to Change
Day 4: Sexercise #4: Developing Your Sexual Voice
Day 6: Sexercise #5: Sexual Initiation

WEEK TWO: Creating Intimacy
(All sexercises in chapter 5)
Day 1: Intimacy Quiz: Take quiz/compare scores
Day 2: Sexercise #6: Sexual Turn-ons/offs
Days 3-7: Sexercise #7: Playing Together
All Week: Sexercise #8: Kissing Exercise

WEEK THREE: Creating Passion
Day 1-5: Sexercise #9 NST: A Touching Exercise (chapter 5)
Day 6: Sexercise #10: Intimacy Over Time (chapter 5)
Day 7: Sexercise #11: Your Sexual Cycle (chapter 7)

WEEK FOUR: Creating Sexual Connections
Day 1-5: Sexercise #9: A Touching Exercise (chapter 5)
Day 6: Sexercise #12: Creating Sexual Transitions (chapter 7)
Day 7: Sexercise #18: Caring Behaviors (chapter 10)

After completing all the exercises above, practice maintenance sex (chapter 7), at least twice, with each of you initiating it once. Initiate maintenance sex after you finish the first 12 sexercises.

BEYOND THE TEN MINUTE SEXUAL SOLUTION

Many couples who have worked with the Ten Minute Sexual Solution for just one month are really happy to experience changes in their intimacy and sex life, including changing their sexual frequency after the first month. Usually, doing the homework starts off awkwardly, with discomfort and some discouragement at how long it takes to reconnect as a couple. It is like riding a bike. At first it feels very awkward, but with practice, it becomes natural. Know that it takes time, and give yourself a month, working on your relationship a tiny bit every day. Don't worry about having sex or increasing your sexual frequency right away.

After you have finished all the exercises at least once, then you can work on maintaining a new intimate and sexual relationship. To maintain and continue to grow in your relationship, the following is recommended, for 10 minutes a day, for at least a few months. If your relationship gets off course, get back on track by spending 10 minutes a day on these sexercises.

TEN MINUTES A DAY TO MAINTAIN INTIMACY AND SEX

1. Practice sexercise #7 at least once a week (10–30 minutes).
2. Practice sexercise #9 at least once a week (30 minutes).
3. Keep kissing on a daily basis (1 minute a day).
4. Practice sexual transitions (10 minutes or less).
5. Negotiate for maintenance sex to add to your usual lovemaking (10 minutes each time).

After trying all of the sexercises in the one month program once or twice, you many find that one or another of the homework assignments works well for you as a couple to renew your intimacy and/or sexual feelings. If you find something that works well for you, remember to repeat it, continue it, and make it a part of your weekly life. For example, the non-sexual touching exercises can be used as foreplay throughout your relationship. The kissing exercise might be something you would like to continue on a daily basis, but it might not be something one or either of you really enjoys at all. Maintenance sex might work very well when it only includes one or two sexual interactions that you enjoy, but not for having sexual intercourse. Find what works for you as a couple, and make a commitment to make it a part of your life.

Some couples find it difficult to complete assignments, finding out they have communication problems, sexual desire problems, or other sexual problems, such as an inability to have orgasms or premature ejaculation. Discovering and dealing with these problems are more complex and will require additional "homework" to solve the problem. These sidelines may take you off course from your immediate goal, but while it may take longer to resolve some problems, identifying and working on specific difficulties will take you closer to your goal of having an active and healthy sex life. In addition to the exercises listed in the one month program, the book contains several other exercises and tips for couples to improve their intimacy and sexual relationship. Most of these exercises are found in chapters 8 to 10. These sexercises are targeted for men and women with specific sexual growth areas, such as how to have a "G-spot" orgasm. Couples can use these individually, as needed.

GETTING OFF TRACK OR SEXUAL AVOIDANCE?

Now, keeping it real, most couples DO get off track from doing their homework and exercises every day. I suggest that couples consider taking two hours a week for their relationship or marriage, especially if doing daily assignments is impossible due to two people working different shifts, traveling in one's job, or going through your child's baseball season. Unfortunately, many couples who do make a commitment to work on their relationship, even for 10 minutes a day, somehow find it difficult to make the time for each other. As a sex therapist, I have heard every possible reason, some reasonable, and some unbelievable. Unreasonable excuses are often sexual avoidance.

Reasonable excuses:
- "My mother had a heart attack and I was in the hospital all week."
- "I was in a car wreck, broke my leg, and was recovering all week."
- "I had to leave town last week and didn't get back in until last night."

Sexual avoidance:
- "We didn't even see each other this week! [Although we slept in the same bed every night.]"

- "We were too busy to do the homework."
- "We had company over and never got 10 minutes alone."

If you can't find 70 minutes a week to spend time with your loved one, then you are not trying to make time for your relationship or marriage, or you are avoiding each other and closeness that might lead to sex. People spend more than 70 minutes a week watching commercials. In fact, the average American spends 4 hours a day watching TV! You might have a very good reason for avoiding closeness, which is addressed in the last chapter. If you haven't read it, review chapter 2 on sexual power struggles, including sexual avoidance. If you are having trouble making time to do the exercises together, one of these things is usually happening.

- You are simply out of the habit of making time for each other, allowing work and children and life to take over your love life. If you are out of the habit, you need to refocus your commitment on making new routines and rituals for your relationship. Turn off the TV, cut back your 70-hour work week, turn off the computer, put the kids to bed on time, make yourself an "adult-centered family," set boundaries with your family and friends, and do what you did so naturally when you were a teenager: Simply be together and forget everything else for an hour or two a week.

- If you must, to create time for your relationship, at first, take time off work, such as a day or a weekend, to begin to be together and focus on your relationship. Stay at home while the kids are in school or daycare or even leave town for a night or two. Get away from your normal routine to plan for a new routine—and life!

- You might be avoiding doing the homework because you are afraid you'll end up in a fight or that it will be uncomfortable. You might question your commitment or your belief in change. Are you thinking, "We've been there, done that! We always fight or feel awkward and nothing changes anyway." One of the first steps is to make a commitment to change—at the same time, together. At least try the second week of intimacy exercises, to see if good feelings fly and if you can reconnect as intimate friends. If you're afraid of conflict, go to chapter 6, and learn how to fight right. You may think it's strange to have a chapter on fighting in a book about sex, but believe me, this is a major problem for couples. You have to learn to deal with disagreements to get past problems, resentments, and fears of moving forward, as a couple.

- You're still engaged in a sexual power struggle (see chapter 2) and one or both of you is avoiding sex. Work to break out of your sexual power struggle by taking a sexual break (see sexercise guidelines above), then doing the first 2 to 3 weeks of sexercises, taking 10 minutes at a time. Start by changing your sexual communication, then work on creating intimacy in your relationship before working on your sexual relationship.

The Ten Minute Sexual Solution is a powerful 30 day program to help most couples who would like to have a more active and fulfilling sex life and who have a little motivation, but not much time, to change and find more sexual pleasure in their lives. You can work the program week-by-week or by trying each sexercise at your own pace, but remember that each set of sexercises builds on the other, and you have to have the foundation of communication and intimacy to be successful with sex therapy. Making a commitment for a month or two months, taking just 10 minutes a day to do it, will give you a goal to keep your relationship moving ahead, giving you hope for change. First, learning to communicate about sex is essential to managing sexual differences and bridging sexual gaps, to learn to enjoy more frequent, satisfying sexual relationships. The next chapter shares the secrets of sexual communication, to allow couples to create a foundation of emotional intimacy and change their sexual relationship, too. In 10 minutes a day, you can get started on learning sexual communication and developing a sexual voice—for life!

CHAPTER

4

Secrets of Sexual Communication

Do you talk about sex? With your lover, that is. Often, when couples come to sex therapy, they feel awkward, embarrassed, and nervous talking about sex or even saying sexual words. Astonishingly, many couples have never talked directly about their sex life with their partner. The truth is, many couples really don't talk openly about how they feel about sex, or what they want before, during, or after sex, making it very difficult for individuals to get what they want.

You can begin to change your sexual relationship by changing your sexual communication, in and out of the bedroom. This chapter will help you learn to talk about sex, and how to be understanding and accepting of each other in order to make the beginnings of a sexual connection possible. In just a few minutes a day, you can begin to share your deepest thoughts and feelings about what you want.

Dr. Darcy's Formula for Successful Sexual Communication

Do you want to instantly change your communication forever? It doesn't take a lifetime or even 10 minutes to learn one secret that can change how you relate to your partner and to each other. The secret is acceptance. In an instant, you will learn that if you are simply accepting of your partner—and tell them—by communicating acceptance, you can change your relationship, almost overnight.

> ### The Formula:
> ### Self-disclosure + Acceptance = Intimacy

Becoming sexually intimate with someone requires first being comfortable with sharing openly about yourself, which requires self-disclosure. Ongoing self-disclosure requires acceptance, if you are going to feel close as a couple. The more you share, the closer you will feel, IF—and that is a big if—you feel embraced when you share your innermost secrets about yourself, your family, your relationships, and your sexuality. Of course, feeling accepted affects whether or not you will use your sexual voice, or even want to talk to your partner, so it is very important for you to work on being accepting, not rejecting, when your partner shares sexual communications.

> ### "We have a communication problem."

Most couples come into therapy saying they have "communication problems." As a therapist, I have found that the very few people actually have communication problems.

> ### The biggest communication problem is: One person doesn't like what the other person says.

That's right! The problem is not communication, it's dealing with what is being said. People don't like it, and then they fight about it. If you have repeated problems with fighting, chapter 6 can help you work on resolving conflicts. For now, understand that acceptance is very important in the formula for sexual communication. Consider the differences in the following communication:

> Jayne: Sweetie, do you want to go have Mexican food for dinner?
>
> Laurel: (ACCEPTING): No, not really, but thanks for asking, I'd rather just eat at home.
>
> OR—
>
> Laurel: (UNACCEPTING): UGH! NOOOO, I do NOT want to eat Mexican food again. That is ALL you ever want to do, eat fattening Mexican food. Gross!

It is so easy, in the course of a day, after you have been together or married a long time, to simply communicate in non-accepting, even hostile ways toward each other. This style of communication can become almost automatic, gradually creating distance in a relationship over time. Think about the way you talk to each other on a day-to-day basis. Is it accepting? Are you kind? Or have you gotten into a routine of saying exactly what you're thinking, acting rude and hostile, without using a loving filter in your communication?

The great part of acceptance is that everyone wants it: They want to be liked for who they are, they don't want to change, and they want to feel loved like they felt at the beginning of the relationship, in that state where everything they did and said was great! In the beginning of a relationship, love is "blind," and people focus on the positive aspects of a person, completely loving them as if they were perfect, ignoring faults. Later in a relationship, people often focus on the problems and ignore the positive aspects. If you want to open up communication, start focusing on your partner's good aspects; be accepting and approving of them, for a change. Remember the admiration you once had for your partner and show it through acceptance.

Of course, if there are major problems with liking and accepting your partner, go to chapter 6 on learning to fight and resolve conflict. Or if there are addictions or abusive behaviors occurring, those can't be accepted either, and you will need professional help. But when it comes to everyday communication and communications about sex, practice being loving, which means practice focusing on the good things in your partner, being tolerant of faults, and accepting them for who they are, without nit-picking their bad qualities. Over time, who wants to have sex someone who always criticizes you?

YOUR BASIC COMMUNICATION TIPS

Start with the basics: Communication requires talking and listening. I've got a great homework exercise below that will give you each plenty to talk about. But you will not do ANY communicating if you don't listen to each other. Sounds simple, right? **Listening is not the hard part: NOT interrupting is the hard part!** And avoiding interrupting with rejecting, judgmental, and blaming statements seems to be the very hardest part.

One of the reasons many couples need to pay the big bucks to a sex therapist is because they cannot do what is stated in the last paragraph. Nope, they just can't do it. Partners interrupt each other, correct each other, accuse each other of lying and exaggerating the truth, tell each other they are full of bologna, don't want to listen to anything they are doing wrong, and are too busy thinking about how to respond to all the "lies" they are hearing and ways to blame the other person for the problem to really, truly hear what is being said and accept any of it as true.

In a therapist's office, the therapist will make each person tell their *perception* of the problem, one person at a time. If someone interrupts, the therapist will tell them to stop interrupting and let the other person finish. If that someone has a huge problem with interrupting, it is often because they are so angry when they think the other person is lying or exaggerating that they feel they must correct them and tell their side of the story. Sometimes a problem with interrupting can mean more serious things; perhaps one person is controlling, very inpatient, very upset about a particular issue, or has an anger problem. Here are some basic tips on open communication.

TEN MINUTE TALKING TIPS

Talker:

1. If you are the talker, don't lie and don't exaggerate.
2. If you are the talker, start your story with, "My perceptions are that I…" or "I think I…." Avoid using the word YOU. For example, if you think you aren't getting enough sex, you say, "I feel like I don't get enough sex," as opposed to "You're always rejecting me sexually."
3. The important thing is to avoid blame. The "blame game" will do nothing but break down communication and build negative feelings between you. Avoid blaming statements that automatically put someone on the defensive, such as "You never give me sex; you are such a frigid person. If you won't give it to me, I'll find someone else who will."

Listener:

1. If you can't keep yourself from interrupting because you are so angry about what is being said, use a pen and paper and write down your objections to keep track of them until it's your turn to talk.
2. If you can't keep yourself from interrupting because you disagree with what is being said, use a stopwatch for each of you to talk for three minute intervals. That way, you will get your turn to say what

you think and feel while still giving the other person a chance to have his or her say.

3. If you feel hurt about what is being said, don't shut down and shut up, either. Use your next turn as the talker to say that you're hurt and why. Answer with statements that reflect back what your partner is saying: "Sounds like you are feeling _____," "I'm wondering if you feel _____," "I understand that you are thinking _____," to show you are listening.

4. Try to be sympathetic, and put yourself in her shoes to understand how she feels.

Work very hard on listening and trying to be accepting, to really get the communication going. Remember, when people are dating, they are talking constantly because there is much more acceptance than rejection.

If you've been harsh, judgmental, or blaming toward each other, it will take time and acceptance to trust each other and open up again

BEING JUDGMENTAL AND BLAMING—AN EXAMPLE:

BLAMING:

CHRIS AND JAMES

Chris says: "James, I feel like I don't get enough foreplay with sex."

James: "Chris, that's not true at all, I almost always give you oral sex before we have sex!"

Chris: "Yeah, sure, you don't even kiss me, you practically rip off my underwear, and then go straight for sex...I hate it!"

ACCEPTING:

Chris: "James, I feel like I don't get enough foreplay with sex!"

James: "Really? I thought that I was giving you foreplay when I give you oral sex before sex."

Chris: "Yes, you are always considerate of my having an orgasm first, but really, I'd like to have more kissing and touching before you give me oral sex."

James: "Okay, sure, I could do that more, that's no problem. I guess when I see you get undressed, I just get excited and I want to go straight for sex!"

Chris: "I know, but I think I would enjoy making love a lot more if we would just make out longer first."

James: "Okay, but sometimes, would it be okay if I can just skip the foreplay and go for it?"

Chris: "Sure, we can do that once in a while, just for you, but I'd like to do it just for me sometimes, too!"

If you start to get into fights and can't seem to get very far, despite repeated attempts at stopping and starting over again, I strongly recommend that you read chapter 6, which has very specific techniques for how to fight and resolve conflicts that most couples will find helpful, if not essential, to communication problems.

THE SEX TALK

Every couple needs to take time to have "the talk." Yes, the sex talk, for adult couples. If you have a low sexual frequency marriage or relationship, you have probably had *many* talks that didn't go anywhere. This talk is different. This talk is not about the problem—it's about the solution.

If you're the person with the higher sexual desire, there is a 99.9 percent chance that you will be initiating any conversation about sex, right? The lower-desire person often wants to avoid any type of sexual conversation, or anything that might lead to sex. Yet, if you're the lower-desire person who is worried about sex, sexual pressure, and what to do about it, initiating the talk is likely to be easier because your partner is more likely to be open and receptive. Just tell them up front: This is not a sexual invitation!

The talk is about being sexual partners, being marriage partners, and working together as a team to address and change your sexual relationship. Just like anything else in your marriage that needs discussion and joint decision-making, so does your sexual relationship. The talk requires that each of you communicate about what you want sexually, how you feel, what you think your partner wants, and to make a commitment to each other to work on your sexual relationship. But first, you'll need some guidance on how to make it work differently this time.

THE SEXUAL PANDORA'S BOX

For some couples, getting started is one of the biggest challenges to sexual change. Bringing up the subject of sex can be pretty difficult and downright scary, since people fear an unpredictable or rejecting response from their partner. Before you picked up this book, it is highly likely that you've already had one or more anxiety provoking or hotly contested arguments about sex. In fact, maybe you're certain what the response will be—not pretty, not funny, or not welcome. You might be afraid of opening the sexual Pandora's box.

Talking about sex can open the door to a lot of problems from the past, worries about the future and your relationship, and concerns about what kind of new demands and pressures might be put on your future relationship. Bringing up the subject of sex—especially when it has been difficult or a source of conflict, fighting or avoidance—is often very hard to do for the closest of couples. In fact, some of the nicest couples avoid talking about sex because they don't want to hurt each other's feelings, even more than they want have sex. Remember, for those individuals with lower sexual desire, it is just as emotionally difficult to talk about sex because of guilt or a fear of sexual pressure as it is for the higher desire person who is frustrated with sexual dissatisfaction. So here are some tips on how to get started:

TEN MINUTE TIP: HAVING THE SEX TALK

- Do give each other permission to talk about sex, without being blamed or judged or ridiculed. Make a promise not to bring up sexual secrets and throw it up in someone's face later, especially publicly.
- Do act loving and accepting, the opposite of judgmental and angry.
- Don't make threats about your relationship or blackmail your partner into reading this book by using the "D word" (divorce).
- Do invite your partner to start by trying just one or two of the exercises
- Don't start with sexual exercises. Start with exercises that involve talking and intimacy, like those in this chapter.
- Don't be afraid of the time for the "homework." Most exercises take 10–15 minutes—and the homework from a sexual self-help book is a lot more fun than assignments from high school or college.

SEXERCISE #1

THE SEX TALK

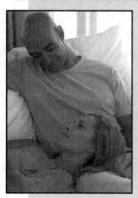

You can begin your sex therapy program with the sex talk. This talk is different than your past talks about sex: It is about the sexual solution, not the sexual problem. To keep your sex talk focused on solutions, not problems, have your first talk limited to the topic of reading this book. Start by talking to your partner, using the sexual communication formula and the 10 minute tips on "having the talk", about why you bought the book. Your talk is not about solving your sexual problems; instead' it is an invitation to begin to talk about wanting change in your intimate and sexual relationship. Keep your talk positive, making a brief statement of how you would like your relationship to be, not how you have experienced it in your past. Invite your partner to read the book, starting with the section that was written just for them, either the higher- or lower-desire partner, in chapter 1. If you have read the book all the way through, highlight one or two concepts that you believe your partner would relate to, such as developing a sexual voice or understanding differences in sexual desire. Let your partner know that this talk is the beginning of many "sexercises" you can try together. Limit your first talk to a maximum of 10 minutes of talking each, remembering this is just the beginning of your sexual communication.

YOUR SEXUAL VOICE

The next step in sexual communication is to develop your sexual voice, whether you're a man or a woman. What's a sexual voice? Your sexual voice is saying what you really think and feel about who you are and what you want, sexually speaking. Having a sexual voice means that you can verbally express your sexual thoughts, feelings, and desires about and for sex. The goal in developing your sexual voice is to feel *comfortable* saying what you want or don't want sexually.

SEXERCISE #2

SEXUAL LANGUAGE

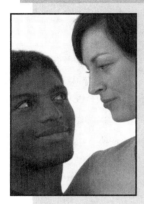

To talk about sex, you need a sexual language. Different people use different words for sex. Some people completely avoid saying the words, so they avoid talking specifically about what they want or think about sex. In this sexercise, you will take 10 minutes to discuss what you like sexual parts and sexual acts to be called.

For example, some people prefer to call a man's penis "a penis." However, most men do not use the word "penis," and they might use another word, such as "dick." Some people might feel turned off or offended if their partner referred to his penis as "my dick." You need find out what your partner calls his penis, or if he has a specific name for it, such as "Henry" (a lot of guys name their favorite part). Discuss what you like to call your parts, and what you call specific sexual acts, such as intercourse, oral sex, sex with a hand, ejaculate/ejaculation, and masturbation. Tell each other what words or phrases you feel comfortable with and what words may be a turn-off (or turn-on!). You certainly don't want to ask someone to go "have sex," or say "I want to hit that" when they prefer being asked to "make love," or you might not get to the lovemaking. Simply focus on sharing sexual language; later, you will talk more about your thoughts and feelings about sex. Remember the first rule of sexual communication: Be ACCEPTING!

YES AND NO

Once you have decided what sexual language you feel comfortable with, the next two words to learn to say are "yes" and "no."

You can't say YES to sex unless you can *really* say NO to sex.

Think about that. If you want to say yes to sex, you really have to be comfortable with saying no to your sexual partner. Being *able* to say no means being comfortable and okay with disappointing your partner and not feeling guilty about not being in a sexual mood or ready for sex. If you can't really say no, without feeling you have to say yes or caving in to sexual pressure, it is not a true "yes": it is being sexually passive, submitting to sexual demands, or sometimes emotional coercion.

For the lower-desire person, giving in to sexual demands usually means you have sex when you don't want to, to please your partner. For the higher-desire person, giving in to sexual demands usually means that you don't ask for what you want. In chapter 7, we'll talk about how to manage differences in sex drives and creating sexual accommodation to work toward meeting everyone's sexual needs, but first, you have got to start being honest with each other about who you are and what you really want. Let me give you a preview of a new sexual script, using "John and Carolyn" as an example.

> John: (coming up behind Carolyn and putting his arms around her waist) Hi, girl, how're you doing tonight? (He kisses her on the back of her neck).

> Carolyn: (sighing deeply while she washes the dishes, her hands too wet to push him away) Not that good, I'm exhausted. Work was so hard today and it sucked the energy out of me!

> John: (continuing with his kisses on the back of her neck) I'm so sorry you had a hard day. Why don't I finish the dishes for you later and you come and sit down on the couch, while I give you a foot rub?

> Carolyn: Forget it! I know you won't do the dishes, they'll be here in the morning, and all you want is sex! I'm so tired, I don't know if I'll have the energy to undress, and I don't want to have sex, not tonight. I know…it's been days since you've gotten

some and you're trying to get me in the mood, aren't you?

John: Okay, okay…it's true, I'm horny as hell, and I would love to have some sex…but really, I know you're beat. I promise I'll do the dishes before the cockroaches attack the kitchen in an overnight takeover, and I really just want to help you relax…by giving you a foot rub.

Carolyn: (looking John straight in the eye) Really, you'll get the dishes done?

John: I promise!

Carolyn: But this IS a ploy for sex, right?

John: Yes, I want to have sex, but NO, there is no sexual expectation, no strings attached, I just want you to feel good and relaxed. I'll even heat up the massage oil and give your soles a hot oil rub down.

Carolyn: Okay, cool…let's go!

USING YOUR SEXUAL VOICE

John and Carolyn were very straightforward about their desire or lack of desire for sex. Carolyn understood John's non-verbal communication, of hugging and kissing her, as well as his offers for dishes and a foot rub, as starters for sex. John was trying to ask lovingly for sex, and even get his wife in the mood for sex. Then, both of them used their sexual voice and said EXACTLY what they wanted and didn't want. John didn't get a commitment for sex, although Carolyn might change her mind after she relaxes and rejuvenates with a foot rub. At least Carolyn doesn't have to feel as much sexual pressure because she already told John she wasn't in a sexual mood. An important step in the Ten Minute Sexual Solution is having a sexual voice and becoming comfortable and safe in stating how you feel about sex, especially saying yes and no.

Your Sexual Voice: A Sexual Communication Exercise

Developing your sexual voice is essential to having a great sexual relationship. Of course, there are other components to a relationship that must be attended to: the secrets of safe sexual communication, and increasing intimacy and resolving conflicts. Nevertheless, one of the first secrets of sexual communication is simply being able to say what you want *during* sex. Some of you have no problem saying what you want, while many of you talk very little during sexual interaction. For those of you who can share with each other every detail of your sexual thoughts, feelings, and fantasies, right down to the moment of "I'm coming!" all the way to asking after sex, "So how was it for you," you can skip this exercise. For everyone else, try this exercise to improve your sexual voice.

TEN MINUTE TIPS FOR USING YOUR SEXUAL VOICE

- **Practice sharing how you are feeling sexually**, and where you are at with sexual desire on a regular basis, using the number rating scale in Sexercise #3. Check in with each other frequently, at least a couple of times a week.
- **Remember the phrase: "Higher, Lower, Faster, Slower."** This an easy rhyme to remember, when you are thinking about, "So what am I supposed to say in bed?" You don't say these all at once, you say which one is necessary and needed at the time.
- **Scream or moan.** Try it, you'll like it. Let your voice release your natural feelings. If you're worried about noise and privacy, use a pillow or a noise buster, such as music or the TV.

SEXERCISE #3

DEVELOPING A SEXUAL VOICE

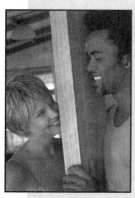

The goal of the sexercise is to tell each other how you feel about having sex, at any given time. Each of you will ask the other person, simply "Are you interested in making love?" (Or having sex, or whatever language you have decided to use for sexual activity). First, say yes or no, and mean it. Next, rate your sexual need or desire and communicate it, using a number scale from one to five. Five is high. Let each other know, "Yes I'd like to make love, but it is no big deal, I can wait a day or two, I'm at a two." Or, "Hey, I am really desperate and needing to have some, I mean, I want to make love with you! I'm at a FIVE!" or "No, I'm not in the mood at all, I'm at a one." For this exercise, simply practice asking each other whether you are interesting in making love, and on what scale. Agree to use this scale of desire to help your sexual communication and begin to use your sexual voice. At this point, don't worry about talking about your specific sexual problems, or initiating sexual activity, simply agree to practice communicating how to rate your sexual needs or desire numerically, without analyzing or judging each other. Remember, communicating your sexual desire does not imply sexual demands. Learning to negotiate with each other about sexual activity is discussed in chapter 7.

- **Finish with:** "Yes, I'm done," or "No, I want to keep going!"
- **Speak up about your likes and dislikes,** regardless of your fears of rejection. To be yourself sexually, to be a part of your sexual relationship, work on developing your sexual voice!

SEXUAL COMMUNICATION AND THE SEXUAL RULES

Sexual communication is difficult for most people. First, as you probably know by now, it is hard for many people to talk about sex. For those of you who were raised in sexually conservative families or with conservative religious training, just saying sexual words can be difficult, let alone talking about a sexual problem. Practice will help and developing trust in your communication will help more. Keep working at it. Second, sexual communication is difficult because most people, both men and women, feel very defensive and self-conscious about sexual performance. No one likes to be criticized or told they aren't doing something right or enough or too long. When it comes to sex, it is a very personal matter and often a performance issue, and people don't want to feel like a failure.

> **Remember, sex is a private act that is special because it is only shared by two people: YOU TWO.**

Develop trust that your sexual communication is private, and what you decide between two consenting adults is okay. In reality, are only three major rules about sex.

SEX RULES!
- First, get permission for sexual touch.
- If someone says no, you stop!
- If there is pain, stop.

Those are the sexual rules, folks! Anything else you two decide between you is really okay, and there's rarely anything to be self-conscious or embarrassed about. For many sex therapists, the first part of the providing therapy is just telling people what is normal and okay and that you are not perverted or weird for thinking, feeling, and wanting the things you do. Of course, there are exceptions to the third rule, for those people who practice sado-masochistic behaviors, but that is beyond the scope of this book.

With love and acceptance, you can develop trust. With trust, you can each open up and self-disclose more and become more intimate with each other. When you can share more of your thoughts, you can move on through each step or at least many of the steps toward solving your sexual problems and increasing the pleasure in your physical relationship.

MAKING SEX A PRIORITY: SPECIAL COMMUNICATION

Most couples in long-term relationships have made a commitment to one another to be monogamous sexual partners, through marriage or a personal dedication and pledge. When two people marry, they make a commitment to be sexual partners for life. If you're married, remember your vows to each other: to have and to hold, from this day forward, until death do you part. Now, to experience change in your relationship, you need to communicate about renewing your commitment to make intimacy and sexuality a priority for your relationship. Accept and understand that a commitment will involve time and effort (just 10 minutes a day), without any guarantees for change.

If your partner will not make a commitment toward working on your sexual relationship, try making an invitation to work on your intimacy and/or communication. Working on the first three steps of the Ten Minute Sexual Solution may seem a lot less threatening than working on your sex life, at first. If your or your partner has absolutely no motivation to make any type of commitment to work on your relationship, or feels quite strongly against making such a commitment, it is possible that you have a serious underlying relationship problem, a medical problem, or a sexual problem, such as one person experiencing painful sex (see chapter 2). There may very well be an important and good reason for not wanting to make a commitment toward sexual change in your relationship, and this reason should be taken very seriously. If an invitation to make intimacy or sex a priority fails, it is recommended that you seek professional help from a marriage and/or sex therapist prior to continuing, or you may make your problem worse. A therapist may help you identify an underlying problem, but until it is identified by one or both of you and you can freely make a commitment together toward change, do not continue with sexercises.

SEXERCISE #4

MAKING A COMMITMENT TO CHANGE

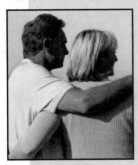

A major step to solving your sexual problem is to create an agreement to work together. You need to agree on three things to set forth your intentions, before you can continue:

1. Make a commitment to work on your sexual relationship together, devoting at least 10 minutes a day, every day, for one month.

2. Start communicating about sex. Practice acceptance; avoid blame.

3. Stop avoiding the problem. No excuses.

You can make a verbal agreement to set forth your intentions and commitment to work on your sexual relationship, but I strongly suggest that you make out a *written* agreement. Take five minutes to write it, sign it, and give it to each other to make your agreement more formal, as well as intimate, using your own words.

Make your written commitments a gift to each other. Some couples have used this exercise as an opportunity not only to make a commitment, but to write a letter of love to each other. Do what feels right, but get each of the three agreements in your letter. Remember, you do not have to agree on specific changes; you only have a willingness or desire to change your relationship.

Here are examples of letters of intent and commitment.

I, Claudine, agree to stop blaming you for my problem, Derek. I will listen to what you have to say, and I will talk to you about how I feel about our problem, as long as you aren't putting all the blame on me, either. I will agree to spend two hours a week, just for working on our sexual and intimate relationship, no matter what, without giving excuses about being too tired, or that it's tax season, and giving us that time as a couple, as an important priority in my life.

I, Derek, agree to stop blaming our sex problem on only you, and to look at our problems as a couple, too. I will agree to start listening and talking, not yelling, about sex. I will agree to spend two hours a week to work on our sex life, even if that means we're not actually having sex, but that we're working on it together because, Claudine, I love you!

SEXUAL INITIATION

Who starts sex? When? Why? How? Sexual initiation is a very important part of a sexual relationship. Communicating about when you want to have sex, when you don't, and how to start sex together as a couple is very important to having an active sex life.

In the beginning of relationships, most couples say, "Well, we both just kind of started sex," or "I'm not sure how it happened. One minute we were hanging out and the next, we were having sex." Couples in long-term relationships with active sex lives often have their own personal signature for their sexual initiations, which are often quite sweet and endearing or even quirky and funny. Sexual initiations come in verbal and non-verbal forms. Sometimes the initiation of sex is as subtle as a longer look or a dilation of the eyes, or it can be more direct, such as asking their partner to go to bed with them or make love or just have sex. It can be somewhere between direct and indirect approaches, such as asking someone to take a bubble bath or have a hot oil rub down.

When couples have a low sexual frequency, sexual initiation is often strained or even very difficult, to the point of being as complex as an act of war. Often the higher-desire partners want to initiate sex, and they are the only ones to do so. Yet, when partners are repeatedly rejected, even if it's a mild rejection, they will stop initiating sex and wait for the lower-desire partner to start sex. Waiting for the other partner to start sex can stop sex altogether, because some people are very uncomfortable with initiating sex.

Successful sexual communication involves developing an understanding and sometimes a personal ritual for sexual initiation. The solution lies in each couple openly discussing the subject. Some people, both men and women, always feel uncomfortable starting sex. Some women feel like men should start sex, period. Some people feel they never get a chance to start sex, because their higher-desire partners want it more and they never have a chance to "get horny." Some higher-desire partners may be waiting for their lower-desire partners to start sex because they don't want to be rejected (again), they may realize that their partners are more comfortable being in control of sex, or they are waiting for a window of sexual opportunity to open. Starting sex can become a stand-off, even when both partners want sex. Some couples are waiting until sex happens spontaneously, perhaps like when they were first dating.

The Myth of Spontaneous Sex

Sexual unity happens when both partners begin to claim their own sexual needs and acknowledge the continual needs of their partner, both inside and outside the bedroom. Each person needs to use his or her sexual voice, so you can discuss and decide together what you want emotionally, intimately, and sexually as individuals and as a couple.

"Hey...But...Sex is Supposed to be Spontaneous!"

"I just want sex to be spontaneous!"

"Sex is supposed to just happen!"

"I want sex to be like it used to be when we first got to together!"

"I don't want to talk about when we have sex or negotiate to have sex, that ruins sex for me!"

"I just want to make love to my lover on the spur-of-the-moment, when the mood hits me!"

Really? Sex is supposed to just happen? And that is how it was when you first got together…right?

Even on TV or in the movies, couples who have spontaneous, ravishing sexual moments, throwing themselves in passionate embraces against the wall or onto a bed while tearing off each other's clothing, without saying a word while they kiss deeply and touch every part perfectly—it usually takes two seasons of episodes for made-for-TV love affairs and months of "movie life" for a couple to consummate a sexual relationship! Even on-screen romances that seem to happen in the spur of an intense passionate moment take weeks or years of time to happen *in the context of a relationship* for a climactic 10 minutes of passionate lovemaking!

As with everything else in life, most things that happen *aren't* spontaneous: they are planned and negotiated so they *will happen.* Some people feel that if they have to plan for and talk about sex and negotiate on when and where it happens, it doesn't "count," because it was planned and not spontaneous. Yet, if you look back to the beginning of your sexual relationships, you will see that this was often there to some extent, as well. Most things in life require planning: getting to work, paying the bills, caring for the dog, preparing for the holidays, and getting your hair cut. Would you say that a great haircut wouldn't count just because you had to make an appointment and wait two weeks for it to happen? Or because you had to ask for it to happen? Would you say that your degree in cosmetology or zoology or medicine doesn't count because it took planning? It wasn't spontaneous, was it? Was your last gourmet meal spontaneous? Did that cheapen it or lessen your pleasure in enjoying it? Why would you think that sexuality would be any different?

It might be true that at one time in your life you were much more obsessed with each other and couldn't keep your hands off each other and it seemed like no one really started sex…it just

SPONTANEOUS SEX IS A SEXUAL MYTH!

So when you were 17 and having sex for the first time (like 80 percent of teens), did you just "do it" on your parent's livingroom floor? Or did you have to make some plans to go out, get your homework done, talk about it, discuss birth control, or find a private place to make out, first?

So when you were in college or in your first real job and you were sharing a dorm room or apartment with someone, did you just magically come together as a couple to make love? Or did it take a little planning: getting rid of your roommate, having a plan to accommodate each other's private/sleep/study times, arranging for a time when the two of you were both available and didn't have a test the next day, coordinating work schedules, and basically planning to be together?

So when you were first living together, did you just fall into bed together every day? Or did you STILL have to coordinate your work schedules, plan for privacy because the people who lived below you always heard your bed squeaking, and deal with your everyday lives, too, such as negotiating about housework and managing money, first?

happened! Even if it was after all of the other details of life were arranged, you still ravished each other. The truth is that people are more obsessive and impulsive in the beginning of their relationship. Perhaps you had (or still have, but less often) moments of "spontaneous sex" early in your relationship, like when you landed on the floor of your family room for 10 minutes (or as long as you could take the rug burns) or other marvelous moments of spur of the moment sex. However, for most couples these impetuous interludes of passion fade or diminish in frequency and intensity.

If you don't have spontaneous sex, it doesn't mean that there is something wrong with your sexual attraction or love for each other!

Even though the obsessive feelings fade over time for couples who really still love each other **remember how a brief, intense,**

ten minutes of sexual passion can be fun, fulfilling, and pleasurable. Planned sex and maintenance sex can replace spontaneous sex in the context of a loving relationship for a couple who has a foundation of sexual trust with each other. In fact, maintenance sex can become spur-of-the-moment sex, if you work on the other parts of the Ten Minute Sexual Solution together! *The Ten Minute Sexual Solution* will help you as a couple to create the sexual trust and understanding with each other to lay a foundation for making your sexual relationship happen, even if it happens to exist after your emotional and sexual needs have been nurtured and cultivated.

> For most couples in long-term relationships, the feelings of sexual desire and sexual intimacy have to be cultivated and nurtured to exist.

Plus, couples need to discuss how to start sex and who will start sex to find out how they like to be approached for making love!

SEXERCISE #5

SEXUAL INITIATION

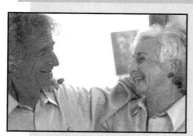

Take 10 minutes to discuss how you like sex to start, or even how you do NOT like to have sexual initiation. Remember that for some people, non-verbal communications work best, such as reaching out to each other in bed and starting by hugging and touching each other. Examples are simply taking someone by the hand to the bedroom without words, asking someone to make love, or creating a "cue word" for wanting sex. You can also use Sexercise #4 to rate your desire for sex in the moment and to find out if your partner is sexually interested. Discuss who you like to initiate sex and how you would like sex to be started. Create your own individual style of sexual initiation.

> **Creating your own sexual signature for sexual initiation is one way to feel more bonded as a couple.**

To use *The Ten Minute Sexual Solution,* you will need learn and practice communicating directly about what you want, what you like and dislike, and when you want to be intimate or sexual or both. Some couples have major communication barriers that need to be broken down before moving on to trying new techniques to change their sexual relationship. If you do, work on resolving them before you continue. Sometimes people don't have a sexual problem but are really struggling with what is actually a communication problem, such as who will initiate sex!

Most couples with low sexual frequency do have some sexual communications problems, but that is not necessarily a barrier to successfully using *The Ten Minute Sexual Solution.* With practice listening and talking, avoiding blame, and being accepting, most people can improve their communication over time. Measure your success with the sexercises in this chapter. Were you each able to speak up and use your sexual voice? Were you able to talk and listen with acceptance to each other's preferences for sexual initiation? Even if you didn't like what you heard, were you able to talk and listen to convey a sense of understanding? If so, you will do well moving on to the next chapter. If not, you may need to learn more about resolving conflicts and addressing major communication problems, which is addressed in chapter 6.

CHAPTER

5

Beyond the Bedroom: What Really Makes a Relationship Work

What really makes a relationship work? Most men are simple: They want more sex, they want to be wanted, and they want to feel appreciated for what they do, but not necessarily in that order! Most women want more emotional intimacy; they want to be made love to all day long, and if you can do that without groping her (after you've taken out the garbage without being asked), then you might find your passionate partner in your bed, but not necessarily in that order, either! This chapter can help both sexes get exactly what they want: to love and be loved...and create a foundation for passion, too!

Let's take a look at marriage, since many people are either married or view marriage as a goal. A great marriage starts with a great friendship, deep intimacy, sharing fun together, special affection, and climaxes in mind-blowing sex! Even if you don't have a great marriage, if you're just looking to get along better and enjoy more lovemaking, start by making love outside the bedroom first!

A great marriage is freedom. Now this may sound like an oxymoron to you. Marriage and freedom, how can they go together?

Some people think freedom means staying single, so you can have as many sexual partners as you would like. But you know that when you're single, you're often sitting around by yourself, lying on your couch, bemoaning the fact that you're lonely! In reality, married partners enjoy much more frequent sex than their single friends[1]. The truth is that a great marriage can be freedom, especially when it comes to sex.

A great marriage is the freedom to love, share, confront, make love, embrace, reject, reaffirm, and return to love again. A great marriage knows that you love each other so much in the long run that you can hate each other in the short run—because it's going to happen. A great marriage gives you the freedom to rejoice, cry, scream, irritate, and love. In a great marriage, you expose your true self, and sometimes it gets hurt hanging out there, but your true self, the real you, also has the opportunity to be loved, and that's when you really feel like you are loved for who you really are, not just when you're dating and someone thinks you're so "great." You never really feel loved until you show them "the real you." When people feel loved for who they are, they can open up and share their most intimate selves, their sexual selves, with trust and love and passion.

The foundation of a great marriage is the foundation for a great sex life. Over the years of marriage, some couples have great marriages, some have good marriages, but in many marriages people grow apart. In fact, they often lose hope and begin to doubt their feelings of love, or they don't feel "in love" with their partner.

> ## In truth, a marriage is a great place to avoid intimacy.

Think about it: If you avoided intimate talks, shared activities, sex, and affection while you were dating, a couple would never stay together! Yet, every day couples avoid and neglect intimacy in their marriages, and some people do it for weeks, months, or years at a time. With today's busy lives, how can a couple whose intimate and sex life has waned or stopped, whether they are married or not, get their relationship back on track?

MAKE YOUR RELATIONSHIP WORK!

First, believe in your marriage or relationship. My husband and I were witnesses to friends sharing marital vows at sunrise on the beach in Folly Beach, South Carolina, on the edge of America, a barrier island off Charleston. The bride's last simple vow to her new husband was to love him "until I take my last breath." Her promise and belief of love was moving. Everyone would like to experience that feeling of hope and love that was shared by this couple on their wedding day. Remember the love you have or once had at the height of your love for each other, even when you have problems in the short-run.

Second, take 10 minutes each day to work on your intimacy. Intimacy is very important outside of the bedroom. Creating intimacy every day is essential for couples to feel close and to stir sexual desire, as well. Assess your level of intimacy in the quiz below. Then read the rest of this chapter to find out how to improve your intimacy and create a foundation of closeness for your relationship or marriage.

Each of the four types of intimacy will be explained in detail in this chapter, including step-by-step explanations on how to improve any single area in your relationship. Just to give you a preview (and some hope), the easiest way to begin to increase your intimacy if you have a very low score is by playing together. It's very hard to start on other areas first. You can't change your past immediately. That happens with trust over time. You usually can't change your level of sex and affection immediately. That's a result of your sharing emotional intimacy first. Sometimes you can work immediately on your friendship, but the easiest way to increase intimacy is by spending time together, doing things with playful

DR. DARCY'S INTIMACY QUIZ

Take a look at your relationship to test how intimate you are together as a couple. Below are four different categories of intimacy that represent different ways couples relate to each other. Rate each of these four areas of intimacy on a scale of one to five, independently from each other, then share your answers and score after you finish. One is the lowest and five is the highest.

FOR EACH QUESTION CIRCLE ONE

Friendship:

1   2   3   4   5

One, we never talk and we're not close. Three, we can talk about almost anything, but we don't always make the time to do it. Five, we are best friends! We can talk about anything!

Sex and Affection:

1   2   3   4   5

One, we never touch and rarely have sex: We're like roommates. Three, we enjoy touching and sex when we have it, which isn't as often as we'd like. Five, we're very affectionate with each other. We're attached at the hip and the pelvis.

Playing Together:

1   2   3   4   5

One, we never do anything together. Three, we have a lot in common, and we do something at least once a week. Five, we're attached at the hip.

Intimacy Over Time:

1   2   3   4   5

One, I don't trust her or him, I always felt let down in the past, and I have a lot of resentments. Three, we haven't been together that long, but so far he's be there for me. Five, we have wonderful memories together and despite our problems, I know she'll always be there for me.

Now add up all four scores to make the total score. Don't cheat...take a risk and rate your relationship individually, then share your scores. Remember: If your scores don't match exactly, scoring can be individualistic and vary, even when you both feel the same way about different categories. What is "2" for one person may be the same as a "3" for another. So when you share your ratings, try not to be defensive, and listen to each other's explanations of how you came to your scores, backing up your reasons with specific examples.

LESS THAN 10 POINTS: TROUBLE AHEAD. If your score is less than 10, your relationship is in major trouble and you need to improve your intimacy, or your relationship will not last. If you are married, it will either fail through divorce or it'll fail through misery. Either way, you do not win at love and sex.

10–15 POINTS: NEED IMPROVEMENT, HAVE HOPE. If it's between 10 and 15, your marriage needs work. You need to strengthen some of the areas of intimacy to have a great marriage. Start with spending time with each other and playing together. Date. Share activities. Laugh. Then work on the homework, especially with friendship first, then affection.

FIFTEEN AND UP: GREAT RELATIONSHIP/MARRIAGE MATERIAL. If your relationship scores over 15, you already have a good to great relationship or marriage and you probably don't *need* this book, but you can benefit from it anyway. You can still have fun with the intimacy exercises, to enjoy feeling closer and the passion of love.

togetherness. The problem with emotional intimacy, if you're like any one of the hundreds and hundreds of clients that I've seen, is that you have a "communication problem" that prevents you from feeling close with each other. If you haven't already read it, go back to chapter 4, to read about sexual communication, but you'll also learn new tips in this chapter. If you have a problem with conflicts and fighting, then read the next chapter to learn to stop arguing and start making love. If you want to increase intimacy in all ways, go ahead and read this chapter and work on the sexercises.

The Four Types of Intimacy

1. Friendship
2. Playing together
3. Sex and affection
4. Intimacy over time

Relationships work when people experience a lot of intimacy with each other. Intimacy makes people feel like they're special people to each other with a special love that's exclusive and different than any other relationship in their lives. Feeling closeness with each other on an everyday basis makes a relationship feel worthwhile and it makes it long-lasting. So let's talk about the four different areas of intimacy.

FRIENDSHIP

Friendship is about emotional intimacy. This comes from being able to talk to each other openly about your feelings and your thoughts, and feeling emotionally supported when you do so. Emotional intimacy can be found by applying the following formula, the same as with sexual communication.

SELF-DISCLOSURE + ACCEPTANCE = INTIMACY

Intimacy comes from the combination of self-disclosure and acceptance, and this means disclosing things about yourself. You start when you're dating, by disclosing or sharing just small daily tidbits of your life, and then you get deeper and more personal about your family, your friends, and your life. Eventually, hopefully, you share and reveal your deepest secrets and your deepest vulnerabilities. You let out one secret at a time, and find out when you reveal these things, whether or not you feel comfortable and accepted.

Self-disclosure may start off with telling each other about your favorite restaurants or music or movies, to share a little bit about yourself. If you feel comfortable, you might go deeper and talk about your past or future dreams. A very deep self-disclosure might be, "I really would like to have a family, and I'm ashamed to tell you that I had an abortion when I was in college." And when there is a response of acceptance, people feel close. This is what true friendship is about. Most relationships start off with true friendship when people have shared simple statements or brief acts that tell about who they are, while waiting to see if they are accepted or even loved for themselves. They may act silly or they may laugh funny, but its most important they feel comfortable.

> ## When you're joined in the joy of who you are, you feel what is called *intimacy*.

Feeling comfortable is key to long-term satisfaction in relationships and marriage. It's more important, in my opinion, than love. People can't define love, but people can define comfort. If you chose marriage with the belief that you would be with this person for the rest of your life, you probably felt comfortable with that person. If you've made a long-term commitment, it is likely you felt comfortable with each other from the beginning. But somewhere along the way that feeling may have diminished. Keeping your friendship is ideal in a relationship, and it makes it an intimate one. Yet, if you forget to remember to share yourselves over time, you will not feel as loved as the years go by.

> ## People "shrink."

If you get criticized, judged, demeaned, ridiculed, or not heard, you will begin to shrink. Your SELF with your partner will shrink. Your sexual self can shrink. The important parts of your self will be hidden or even disappear from your relationship. For example, if you loved playing the piano and your partner hates listening to those "noisy banging keys," you will shut the lid on the piano and let it collect dust. Over the long-run, if you're not accepted in small and big ways, you will shrink; you won't share those parts of yourself, and you will stop being close friends. You need to get back to friendship.

Being emotionally supportive means you can turn to each other to share the joys, sorrows, everyday laughs, and everyday experiences of a lifetime together. If you want to have emotional intimacy, make sure that you have one-on-one time every day, even just 10 minutes a day, for just being friends, being supportive, and helping each other grow, not shrink.

> **The more you share of yourself, the more your true self will feel loved.**

Be sure to make time to have one on one time together for just talking. Turn off the TV and/or the computer to have 10 minutes a day or at least 30 minutes twice a week, to sit together without distractions and pay attention to each other. Find undistracted time to look at each other, listen to each other, and support each other. If you have kids, get them settled into bed early. If you have teens, well, maybe your time needs to be in the morning, or on your lunch hours, or on the weekend when they're sleeping in. Pour a cup of tea, coffee, or even a glass of wine. Turn off the cell phones and house phone. Light a couple of candles, or enjoy the morning light. Start with easy topics, such as work or how your day went. These feelings can be about each other or everyday things that affect your life, such as everyday highs and lows, situations with work, friends, children, church, and family. Being best friends is ideal in a marriage and makes your relationship close. However, even if this is not the case, just being emotionally supportive means you can turn to each other to share the joys, sorrows, and everyday experiences of life together.

If you're not talking now, and you're not even friendly with each other, then you seriously need to ask, do I feel accepted? Do I feel too criticized? Have I shut down? Have I shrunk into a person I don't even recognize with my life partner? If that's the case, friendship and emotional intimacy is what you need to work on. If it's not the case, begin to open up. Take the time, 10 minutes a day to talk, or take one minute a day to call or text message with each other, to communicate and share jokes, share intimate secrets, and be friends.

That's where you start. If all of your talks simply turn into arguments, see the next chapter for learning to fight right.

SEXERCISE #6

INTIMACY EXERCISE: SEXUAL TURN-ONS/TURN-OFFS*

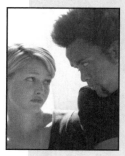

Using the communication tips, talk about your sexual turn-offs and turn-ons. First, take a few minutes to think about and write down your own answers, separately from each other. Be a little descriptive in your answers. For example, don't just write "kissing," write "passionate kissing, French kissing, wet kisses that last at least 5 minutes, while we're hugging each other or only during sex." Or for "oral sex," specifically state what you like, such as: "I love giving and receiving, spitting, not swallowing, one person at a time, no 69!" Take 10 minutes to share your top three sexual turn-offs and turn-ons on your lists. Share answers, one at time, taking turns with each other. Later, you can share more of your lists, when you have 10 more minutes, leaving some of the best for later.

Don't include anything that doesn't involve monogamy, but don't be afraid to say what you really like, unless you absolutely know your partner is against it. The most common line I hear from clients about their partners is: "They'll never change...they'll never do that!" An example is a recommendation for the use of a vibrator for women who are nonorgasmic or not easily orgasmic. While many partners have told me that their partner would never agree to use a vibrator, later most women have changed their mind, only to find out their new toy became one of their favorite turn-ons! Be willing to self-disclose, taking a risk to say what you like and you don't like. Most of the time, as a sex therapist, I see very accepting partners who are excited to hear, "Sure, we can try that!"

*ALTERNATE INTIMACY EXERCISE: DREAMS AND GOALS

If your partner is not ready to talk about sexual topics, but you want to work on your communication and emotional intimacy, use this alternative exercise. Or you can use this at a later time, when you are in the "maintenance phase" of the Ten Minute Sexual Solution.

Talk about your goals and dreams. Share your thoughts about your visions of life, as if money was not an issue. Many couples do not know their partner's innermost hopes and secret desires. Some people think they must shrink or give up their dreams when they make a long-term commitment, marry, or have a family. Create an atmosphere of support by listening, rather than pointing out obvious objections to barriers and problems or even trying to fix a problem. For example, if your partner wants to learn to fly planes, talk about the wonder of flight and the feelings about being a pilot as opposed to how you don't have the money for such a stupid, extravagant expense when you owe $11,318 on only one credit card. Talk about how each of you might one day pursue a part or all of your dreams in your lifetime.

PLAYING TOGETHER

Playing together is having shared activities, common interests, and having fun together. Doing things together and having fun makes people feel closer. Remember what kind of things you did when you were dating? Like going out to eat or watching movies together, or going to the bars and watching bands together. Most married couples stop doing these things because of distractions from work, family, getting older, and getting set in your ways. Most people, when they're dating, go out once or twice a week or every day, but in long-term relationships and marriages it might only be once a month, or it might be three years after your child is born. It's no wonder that most couples feel more in love before they got married: They are having fun playing together!

It's important that each person have his or her own hobbies and interests, but sharing some activities and interests really keeps your relationship strong. If you find that you have no shared time together, then you need to work on developing new interests together as a couple. People change as they grow and as they age and their interests change, too. Even if you had many things in common five, ten, or thirty years ago, these interests might have changed. You need to make a special effort to brainstorm together and find playful and fun things to do together, whether it's going out to eat, traveling, going to church, attending sports events, or even volunteer activities.

A lot of times when I talk to couples I ask, "What'd you do together when you first got together?" They might say, "Well, we met at school and we used to like to go to clubs and listen to bands, and then we'd like go hang out with friends, drink and stay up till 2:00 or 3:00 in the morning talking." Then I ask "And what do you do now?" And the response is, "Well, we don't drink anymore and we don't go to bars, our friends are busy with their jobs and kids, so now we stay home and don't do anything together. I mean, maybe we watch TV, but sometimes we're in separate rooms, where I'm watching TV and he's on the computer, and we're doing different things." There's no shared time together. There's no companionship. As couples grow up together, as a relationship continues and grows, people have to develop these interests together.

Couples need to work on creating new interests and activities as their relationship and personalities change and grow, to share time together. You can have a brainstorming session and think about taking up scuba diving together, or learn how to cook and invite people over, or simply have fun watching your favorite TV show on Thursday night. Some couples think that spending time together means planning a weekend out of town once a year or so. If you wait until you can line up a babysitter and find the weekend of your dreams, you might be waiting too long. Find things to do together around the house, on ordinary days, to simply laugh and play together. Finding things to do together and cultivating common interests will make you feel more intimate and close.

SEXERCISE #7

PLAYING TOGETHER

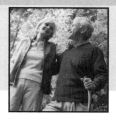

Your homework is to find TWO shared activities to do each week: one that each of you thinks of individually, but both of which that you can agree on doing. Do NOT plan to do WORK (like paint the kitchen): This is for playful fun! A typical activity might include dinner or a movie, and that might be as exciting as it gets. This may be enough, but having a shared interest or hobby together beyond this will draw a couple closer. Intimacy needs to happen on a daily basis, and shared activities need to happen at least twice a week while you're trying to get things back on the great marriage track and make your commitment worthwhile. It doesn't have to be a "date," just spending time together, like you did when you were first falling in love. Perhaps you both want to take a ride in your car, cook a new dish, stare at a full moon, learn skydiving, take up golf, plan a picnic, go to the beach or mountains for a day trip, buy a new CD and bring it home to listen to (or dance to together). Whatever each of you decides to do once a week, do it without friends, children, or family members. DO take turns with ideas for fun and do things together. Activities do not have to be extensive, such as a long weekend away. Try to think of one activity you can do at home and one outside of your home, too. Creating and sharing activities is the easiest way to increase intimacy in your relationship, even for 10 minutes a day.

SEX AND AFFECTION

Now, most people think of intimacy as: "How much sex do we have?" That's how we measure intimacy: It's a sexual yardstick. But that is not what I'm talking about here. I'm not talking about just sexual intimacy. I'm talking about being affectionate and touching, kissing, and hugging on a daily basis. All of these things are important for a strong relationship and marriage. Even sitting together on the couch and watching TV and holding hands or touching feet across a bed at night can make people feel connected. Sex is one type of physical intimacy, but it's only a small part of the physical intimacy that people crave. People get skin hunger. People need to be touched.

The number one thing women tell me when there's a low sexual frequency in a relationship, when basically everything else is going well, is:

> "I don't want to just go to bed and do my duty. I want him to make love to me all day long, so I'll feel like making love at the end of the day."

Generally, women want physical and emotional attention before they desire making love, while men don't feel they need that as much. There's a gender difference, but there's a solution to the gender difference. It's that you have an understanding that this difference tends to exist, so affection and sex both can have a place in a relationship. Kissing, touching, hugging, and sharing loving feelings together on an everyday basis is an important start to having both partners' needs met in a relationship.

When sex stops, touching stops. When one partner is avoiding sex or doesn't want to have sex as much as their partner, then physical affection and touching becomes very limited, because the lower-desire partner doesn't want touching to lead to sex. To avoid sex, they avoid touching. When the affection and touching subsides, the higher-desire partner not only feels sad about the lack of physical affection, but she wonder if she is loved, wanted, or even attractive to her partner any more.

AN AMAZING DISCOVERY

One of the most amazing discoveries I have made as a sex therapist is how little couples in long-term relationships (more than two years) kiss on a daily basis. I have been totally astonished to find out that the average couple does not passionately kiss...all the time or even on a regular basis. The typical couple gives each other a "peck" good morning or goodbye on the way to work or goodnight at bedtime, but they do not passionately kiss with an open mouth on a daily or even weekly basis. In fact, the majority of couples save deep kissing for making love...if then.

This is so amazing to me! Why don't couples kiss ALL the time? Kissing can be so passionate. When most of us were 16 years old or so, if we had a boyfriend or girlfriend, we were kissing constantly, right? I've even heard of teenage couples puking up excessive beers on a Friday night and deep throating each other again before the night was over. On the other hand, if some adults don't sterilize their mouth in preparation for the once a week, "now-we're-having-sex kiss" (let alone sterilizing other parts of their body), then passionate, sexy kissing is out.

SEXERCISE #8

THE ONE MINUTE KISSING EXERCISE

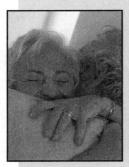

I strongly suggest to every couple that I see that they begin to kiss again, and passionately. Kiss every day for at least one minute, open-mouthed. Hug while you're doing it. Ravish each other's bodies for a minute. Sit on each other's lap. Enjoy being loving and affectionate to each other, with no strings attached. Be passionate and enjoy! Kiss every day for at least one week, but try to keep it up for a month: it's only one minute a day! You might find yourself developing a life long habit of affection and passion.

AND THEN THERE'S: "THE PENIS PROBLEM" (FOR WOMEN ONLY)

Some women complain that when they kiss and hug passionately—I'm talking about one moment of passion here—their male partners get excited and get turned on and, well, they get a hard-on that a woman can feel. And then the woman feels obligated to do something about this "condition." This is, believe it or not, a big problem. I am here to remind all women of some simple but important biological facts concerning "the penis problem."

Men get erections every 90 minutes from the time they are in their mother's wombs, even before they are born, continuing incessantly throughout their lives, ranging from raging hard-ons to only partial erections. The mathematical and biological calculation results in this fact: Your man has had many—thousands and thousands—of unused erections in his lifetime. In your man's early years, this might have been a problem, such as in middle school when those erections appeared out of nowhere and seemed to pop up just before the bell rang, and he had to stand up and publicly move to his next class. However, by the time most men have had a few thousand unused erections, they have learned to manage not using them when they didn't need to. So the moral of this penis problem story is simply this: Tell him you're not interesting in sex, but you just want to let him know how much you love him and want him. You don't have to feel guilty! Go ahead and kiss, and you'll both love sharing the affection!

Reasons for Avoiding Kissing

Most of the time, the reason for not kissing falls into one of these categories, the first being most common for lower-desire partners.

- **Avoiding sex.** "If I passionately kiss him, then he'll want sex." The biggest reason for not kissing is a fear of it being interpreted as a sexual invitation. So people avoiding hugging, touching, kissing, and all sorts of simple physical affections to avoid sex.

- **Hygiene/ germ phobias.** "He has bad breath," or "Ew…I just think of the germs." A small minority of people are germ and body fluid phobics. Not only do these people avoid kissing, but they avoid bodily fluids associated with sexual contact, such as the contact of semen with sex and oral sex.

- **Don't enjoy the way their partners kiss.** Unfortunately, you have to tell your partner, use your sexual voice and say what you like, then practice.

- **Avoiding intimacy.** Some people don't kiss because in reality, they don't want to be that intimate with their partners. For example, prostitutes don't kiss their johns.

- **Being out of the habit.** Some people simple associate passionate kissing with sex and don't think about kissing every day. Yet, when they do start kissing again, these people often enjoy it.

SEXERCISE #9

NST: A TOUCHING EXERCISE

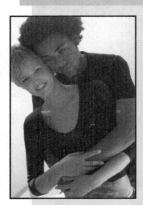

Nonsexual touching (NST) is a type of lovemaking to help partners focus on physical touching and affection without the anxiety, demands and fears of sexual pressure that you may have been experiencing together.

Once a week, *each partner* will initiate NST once with their partner, for 10 minutes. After the first 10 minutes, you will trade places, with the initiator being touched by his or her partner for 10 minutes. When you are the initiator, find a time when you both have 20 minutes of private, uninterrupted time, you are not totally exhausted, and it is not the ninth inning of the World Series. Invite your partner, in your own special way, to go to your bedroom, undress, and enjoy your touching exercise. If one of you feels very uncomfortable with nudity, you can start this exercise by being partially dressed, if this is more comfortable, for the first few times. If you would like to have the lights dimmed, that is fine, too.

The initiator of touching will start, as described below. NST does NOT include touching any sexual parts, hence the word "nonsexual," and, most importantly, you must agree to not have sex afterwards. It is very important that this touching exercise NOT be associated with a demand for sex. It is important that your touching be completely for the joy of touching, with no strings attached. Each partner can enjoy touching each other in any way that he or she would like, such as rubbing the back, stroking hair, touching legs, hands, face, and feet, but not any sexual parts. Sexual parts include the genitals, buttocks, breasts, and nipples. During nonsexual touching, I recommend no talking, except to tell your partner if you are uncomfortable. Your goal as the initiator is to simply enjoy the pleasure of touching and pleasing your partner, in a nonsexual way, without the demands of sex. The partner being touched is to simply enjoy the feelings being touched. Your skin is the largest sex organ, so enjoy sharing giving and receiving the pleasure of its touch.

Important: NO groping. Groping in this exercise will sabotage your Ten Minute Sexual Solution. It is important to share touch that is not sexualized in order to develop trust with touch. Be intimate in your touching, but do not break the rules or you'll lose the value of this sexercise. Enjoy!

INTIMACY OVER TIME

Intimacy over time is about the bond you've created as a couple over time. As you look into your relationship's past, how do you each answer the questions "Has s/he really been there for me?" and "Do I think s/he will be there for me when the going gets rough?" Intimacy over time is about being there for each other and knowing you can count on each other through thick and thin. Generally, the longer you're together as a couple, the greater your bond from time, from trust over time, because the history you share creates a special intimacy. Whether it's sharing births or deaths or job changes or moves, every couple has their own life history they uniquely share with each other, and it makes them feel bonded to each other. This history might include having children together or extended family, a family business, or just growing up together. For some couples who have been together a long time, their history is the strongest component of intimacy in their relationship. Even when a friendship fades, or when sex is less frequent, or a couple has less in common, people stay together because they have a shared past.

For any couple at any stage in their relationship, creating a positive history together is important in creating intimacy. And I'll give you a few hints: First and foremost, you need to be there for each other. I'll give you men an example: You need to be there for your wife when she has your children. Don't order pizza in the delivery room. Make sure you're there as a coach. It's her day, so please her by doing what she asks. You'll hear this birth story for the rest of your life! Make it a good memory.

Women, learn to be supportive to your partner when it's his day. This day may be when they are in the hospital, passing a kidney stone, and they need you to ask the doctor for more pain medication. Or it may be when his mother dies and you have to plan the funeral arrangements, even though his sister should be doing it. You'll hear *this* story for the rest of your life. Whatever the important situation is, be there with love for each other, and you will remember it lovingly.

Same-sex couples have similar important moments, when they need their partners to be there for them. When it's an important holiday and you can't go home with your partner, because the family doesn't accept you, what do you do? Work together to create your own holiday and ritual and family of choice, whether you are together on that day or you agree to celebrate a day later, to have your own special memories and support each other.

For some couples who've been together a long time, there is a strong bond of experiences and intimacy over time. They are each other's family: their past, their present, and their future. Unfortunately, for some couples, even if they've been together for a long period of time, there are milestones when one partner isn't there for the other. For example, I got a call from a client the day after her son was born, who told me, "When I was having the baby, my husband was in a hotel room with his girlfriend, and I couldn't find him to tell him I was in labor." That delivery room story created a very sad history, leaving a deep resentment that eventually led to divorce.

Beyond the bedroom is where the foundation of your sexual relationship is built. A great relationship starts with a great friendship, deep intimacy, sharing fun together, special affection, and climaxes in mind-blowing sex! Couples with sexless relationships have often lost one or more major areas of intimacy in their life. Sometimes the lack of emotional intimacy leads to a loss of desire for sex. For most women and some men, they need to feel close emotionally before they will feel like making love. For some couples, a lack of sexual desire causes sexual avoidance, which will cause emotional and physical avoidance, keeping a distance from behaviors that might lead to sex.

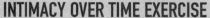

SEXERCISE #10

INTIMACY OVER TIME EXERCISE

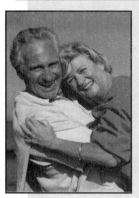

Find a time when you have at least 30 minutes to just sit and talk, without interruptions. (Okay, this one takes more than 10 minutes, but I give you a couple days to work on it!) Recount together the top three times in your lives that you have "been there for each other." Take turns to reflect upon and share your memories of these moments together. Listen to each other with the kind of compassion and love that you remember you once shared. Affirm for each other that you will be there for each other in the future. If you have made mistakes and were not there for each other once or twice, identify specific ways to avoid the mistakes in the future, and then refocus on the memory of the times you *were* there for each other. Make a pledge to communicate to each other that when you do need each other, you can trust and count on each other. Make a promise to be specific about what you want and need, so you can care for each other in the way each of you wants to be loved. Make a pledge to talk to each other when you need each other to develop trust. Make a promise to care for each other in the way each of you wants to be loved.

Whether your sexless relationship is caused by a lack of emotional closeness or your lack of sexual desire caused you to avoid intimacy, regaining your intimacy as a couple is essential to enjoying a loving relationship or marriage. Start with friendship first. Become friends again and talk and play and simply enjoy each other's company, specifically agreeing to remove sexual pressure and focus on your relationship first. Recall your feelings of attraction and admiration for each other. Remember to appreciate each other and really spend time together, even if it is for only 10 minutes a day. For yourselves, your children, and your relationship, rekindle your emotional intimacy, friendship, and affection toward each other. Most importantly: Have fun, laugh, and play again!

CHAPTER

6

Learn to Fight Right: Stop Arguing and Start Making Love

Anger poisons a sexual relationship. Anger is the number one relationship problem that contributes to sexual problems. Anger is not an aphrodisiac, it is a sexual turn-off. Unresolved anger or ongoing anger in a relationship kills sexual desire. While many couples recognize that they fight too much, they don't realize what a huge impact it has on their love life! Women, especially, need to have safety, to feel comfortable with their partners, before they can feel sexual attraction and desire sex. Men often grow quiet and distant when they feel they are being constantly nagged and treated unfairly or unkindly. Learning to communicate and successfully resolve conflicts is very important to allow you to love each other and maintain positive feelings of respect, as well as sexual attraction.

The Ten Minute Sexual Solution will only work if you can learn to fight right and resolve the problems of life together as a couple. Couples whose relationships are long lasting and happy learn to fight right and get over their problems. It doesn't even matter what kind of problems a couple has gone through: They've dealt with births, death, teenagers, car accidents, infidelity, substance abuse, job losses, and many other things. The question is: Do they talk it through? Or eventually "joke through it?" Do they get over a problem, big or small, so they can move beyond it? Or do they at least agree to disagree on a problem that is not solvable, but isn't crucial? In relationships that are dysfunctional, couples get into a fight and problems get swept under the rug, where they remain unresolved. If you never talk about it, you'll never get over it.

> ### Don't push anger under the rug: It usually ends up under the covers.

You may be yelling at each other about how you're supposed to manage the toothpaste in your house, whether you put the cap on or not, or if you squirt it from the middle or the end, whatever. Eventually, you've got to talk to each other about the problem and say, "Look, I prefer the cap on. You don't. Let's have two different toothpastes. Yours will stay on your side, mine on my side, and then let's forget about it." That's a solution. You still haven't solved the problem of not liking the cap lying around the bathroom, or that they have a habit of ruining a tube of toothpaste by squeezing it from the middle, but you've figured out how to deal with a problem that bothers you. For the little things and for the big things, you have to create a solution. Every unresolved argument lays another brick in the foundation of a wall of resentment between you.

> ### Unresolved conflicts create resentment. Resentment turns into contempt. Contempt is the foundation upon which divorce is built.

FIGHTING TO WIN

Learning to fight is one of the most important skills in a happy, healthy, sex-filled relationship. It is an art, an act of maturity, and an essential foundation on which to grow love. Fighting fair ultimately does not mean fighting to win. The moment that you cross that line—from fighting fair to fighting to win—you will lose the argument. People who fight to win often want to control, and they hate the sensation of being out of control. The reality is that when you try to control an argument, you've lost control—it's an illusion. Control is always an illusion. In reality, by fighting to win you just push someone away from you, rather than resolve a problem.

People who fight to win also need to be right. The need to be the only right one goes hand in hand with the blame game: "It's your fault, it's your fault, and it's your fault. If it wasn't for you, there wouldn't be any problems." The blame game is another illusion that people maintain that kills intimacy. Truth be told, sometimes when you're right, that's all you have…your rightness, as if that is the most important thing in the world. But the most important thing is love, and finding a way to love, which is the pathway to making love. You can agree to disagree because you are both individuals with different opinions. There can be differences: There is space between the two of you that allows for individuality. The ultimate goal of the argument is to solve a problem and make new agreements to avoid future problems and live a happy life. Almost all of us can learn to communicate, to fight right, and win in the long-run: to share love and sex.

KAITLYN AND JAMES' STORY

Kaitlyn was 22 and engaged to be married to her boyfriend of two years. She was planning a wedding to take place after college graduation. She came in for counseling because she and her fiancé loved each other very much, had great fun and sex together, but they had a lot of fights—like two or three times a week, almost half of the time they saw each other. Kaitlyn became angry very easily. When she became upset, she would use a loud, piercing, high-pitched voice and begin repeating her side of the story over and over again, interrupting James continually, never listening to him, and insisting on being right and having her way, until he just grew silent and stopped talking to her. Kaitlyn was quite angry that "he would sulk," and wouldn't communicate with her when she was "just trying to talk." Interestingly, she thought he had a communication problem.

Looking at her patterns in resolving conflicts in other relationships, Kaitlyn revealed that when she was in high school, she fought with her mother every single day. Kaitlyn couldn't wait to go to college to get away from her mother. She was so happy she was getting married, so she didn't have to go home after college.

When it was identified in counseling that her style of communicating anger was a form of verbal badgering and unproductive, she replied, "I know, that's the way my father is and my sister is, and I'm just like that, and I'm never going to change." Kaitlyn believed that her learned behavior of getting her way through verbal assaults was okay and justifiable since it was an "inherited trait." Kaitlyn had been told repeatedly by her mother, father, friends, and previous boyfriends that she started fights by yelling, interrupting, badgering, and controlling arguments until she got her way. She had basically learned to have temper tantrums until someone gave in to her because they couldn't stand her screeching! Unfortunately, Kaitlyn saw the resolution of this problem as her fiancé just accepting it because "that's just the way I am."

Kaitlyn came into therapy to try to convince her fiancé that she was right and he was wrong. She was astounding in her resolve that she was genetically programmed to be abusive, which somehow made it perfectly okay.

Kaitlyn had an idea of who she was when it came to her anger, but she did not accept the fact that she had poor skills in communication and conflict resolution, or that she needed to change herself—or could—due to her family legacy. She really didn't see her family legacy as a true problem. In fact, she honored the legacy by acting it out.

Therapy was a true shock for Kaitlyn. She refused to change. She feared if she did, she would lose control and no longer get her way. Kaitlyn did not realize that her idea of control was an illusion, and her fighting to win meant she was going to lose. Kaitlyn refused to believe this and even tried her yelling and screeching routine in my office! After 10 seconds of her screeching, the therapy session was ended. Kaitlyn was told that she could have her temper tantrums outside the office as much as she wanted, but I would not participate in verbal abuse in my office. She left. Her fiancé stayed. He informed me, there and then, that he was breaking the engagement, and then he left. I never saw James again.

Four months after their broken engagement, Kaitlyn called me. No one sympathized with her, not even her father. At first, she decided she was better off without James and his sulky moods. Then she told her parents and her friends to go to hell and that she didn't need them. She maintained her blame game, repeating "It's his fault" for several weeks. After four months of partying, dating other people, and trying to convince herself that she was right and James was wrong, Kaitlyn became depressed with grief over really missing James, whom she loved. She had lost her love under the illusion that by being in control, she would win. She looked in the mirror, realized that what everyone was telling her was right, that she had a problem, and decided to seek individual therapy and learn to fight right.

Dr. Darcy's Ten Rules for How to Fight Right

1. No abuse: no physical abuse, no yelling, no name calling, no cursing
2. Take turns with anger
3. Call a time-out and cool off
4. Do finish a fight
5. No silent violence
6. Do not fight to win
7. Admit when you're wrong
8. Learn to say "I'm sorry"
9. Solve the real problem
10. Take turns being right

1. NO ABUSE: NO PHYSICAL ABUSE, NO YELLING, NO NAME CALLING OR CURSING.
Absolutely no physical aggression, including physical intimidation, like punching holes in the wall or pounding a fist on a table, is acceptable in fair fighting. No yelling, no hitting, slapping, grabbing, or pushing someone up against a wall, unless you don't want to be in a relationship or married anymore.

Many people lose their tempers and yell, just lash out, and are verbally abusive when they get angry. If someone is having a bad day and losing it and starts yelling: STOP! When you yell back, when you start to yell back and forth, everything that you say from that point forward will only be destructive, it is NEVER productive. Think about it…did you ever have anything good come out of a screaming match? I doubt it.

> If someone starts swearing or yelling, stop the fight. Anything said after that will not be productive and is usually destructive.

TEN MINUTE TIP

I'll share a secret with you. If your partner tells you that you are yelling and/or they feel physically intimidated, *they are*. If you are arguing, and they thinks it's yelling or they feel intimidated, YOU ARE YELLING! Although it may not seem intimidating to you, really try to listen to them and change your tone to communicate respectfully. Why would you disagree and argue with someone who is afraid of you? Do you think this person who feels fear will want to make love with you later? No, because love and fear are incompatible emotions to experience at one time. Some people, especially men, do anger like they breathe. They take in a deep breath, yell out what they're mad about, get over their problem, then exhale, change the channel on TV and say, "Hey, what's for dinner? You wanna have sex later?" When men get no response, they justify their anger indulgence with more anger, yelling, "Okay, I got angry!" And women react to the anger outburst with hurt, anger, or fear, still shaking in their boots even later.

Stop calling each other names, including using curse words. The names will be remembered long after a fight—sometimes for years! Listen closely to these words, spoken across from me in my office, from a couple talking about their recent separation.

JOSH AND LILY

Josh: "Why do you want to get a divorce?"

Lily: "I don't know, Josh, it's just so many things we don't agree about and we always fight. And I don't like how you treat me when you get mad."

Josh: "What did I do? What did I say?"

Lily: "I've estimated that over the course of our [six year] marriage, you've called me a bitch about 500 times."

Josh: "But I didn't mean it, I was just angry!"

Lily: "Josh, the sad part is that I believed it, and I think you were right, I was a bitch!"

Josh: "I'm sorry, but I was right, you were a bitch sometimes!"

Lily: "Yep, Josh, you're right, I was a bitch, at least 500 times, to you. And I've decided that you were right, I became a bitch with you. I don't like who I've become. I have to say, Josh, the reason we're separated is because you were so right."

Sadly, Josh and Lily divorced. It was interesting that Lily added up and estimated how many times she was called a bitch, and Josh didn't even disagree! I guess he called her a bitch one too many times. Truthfully, if he had listened to her instead of telling her she was being a bitch, he might have known exactly why she was so unhappy and the real reasons why she eventually left him. Calling someone a name and cursing at them will often end a fight. Lily recalled several times that she tried to talk to Josh about marriage problems and he stormed off saying, "You're such a bitch!" Maybe she was talking to him disrespectfully, but his yelling and cursing at her, then leaving, prevented them from solving the problems. If they had learned to fight right, they might have stayed together. In the end, all Lily could think about was all the times she was cursed at. It cursed their marriage. Stop calling each other names, stop giving empty apologies for it later, and start listening instead.

2. TAKE TURNS WITH ANGER

Think of anger like a vacuum cleaner: Only one person can use it at a time. When you're both trying to grab onto the handle of the vacuum cleaner for control, you only suck the life out of each other. Nothing will suck the air out of a room like shrieks of anger. Learn to take turns with anger. Only let one person be angry at one time. Even if you're mad at the same time, wait your turn. Try to develop the trust in your relationship that each of you will be given your fair share of time to express your thoughts and feelings. Take the time to agree that if your partner is angry, you will listen, even if you disagree with what is being said. If your partner is having a bad day and losing it, let him talk. Don't just yell back.

Take turns with anger, giving each other some space between you for your individual emotions. You don't have to get sucked into your partner's emotions. Work at having "low emotional reactivity," which is caring but not getting carried away by both of your emotions. If you are being yelled at, become very calm and gentle in your speech, be the mature one, be the patient one, be loving, and your partner will likely calm down, too. Being patient, being calm amidst anger: THIS is what people call the "work" of marriage, or long-term committed relationships.

Many people don't listen; they talk over another person, interrupting them, and not allowing them to get a word in edgewise. Some people feel like they have to get angry and yell back to get someone's attention. I've heard many people say, "If I don't yell, they won't hear me or they won't take me seriously." At times, when someone yells at you, for no reason, or for the wrong reasons, or when there is a misunderstanding, it is hard not to feel angry. You can choose not to express your anger, yet. You are an adult, not a child. You can wait to take your turn. Certainly, if your partner is upset, especially if it is over something that is a misunderstanding, try to talk to them to help them calm down. But, if they don't calm down, let them say what they have to say while you wait for your turn. Once your partner knows that you will listen to them, take their concerns seriously, and talk things over, you will both learn that you don't have to yell or get angry to be heard. You will learn that you can wait on anger. If your partner can't stop, or you can't control yourself, or the matter is just so upsetting that you need time to cool off and think, then take a break.

3. CALL A TIME-OUT AND COOL OFF

In the case of physical or verbal abuse, always call a time out. If one person is so upset that yelling starts, call a time out and honor it at all times! When you are just so upset that you can't think straight or talk without yelling, then call a time-out, and give yourself time to cool off. Cooling off your emotions can make talking out problems possible.

TEN MINUTE TIP: TIME-OUT

- Mutually agree, as a couple, to make the "T" time-out sign like a football referee. Respect a call for a time-out! But, don't abuse it and call time-out every time you try to talk, like right after you got the last word.
- Separate and leave each other alone. Don't follow the person and "force them to talk." Take a break, go to the other end of your home, give each other space, and cool down.
- Usually an hour will be long enough for a break. Try talking after an hour. If that isn't enough, try another hour. If that isn't enough, sleep on it and talk the next day.
- If one of you is the type that feels you have to leave the house and take off, agree on this ahead of time. Agree upon a place to go for "time-outs," such as Wal-Mart, a walk around the block, or the local batting cages. Respect each other's wishes against time-out locations, such as a local bar or your blabbermouth sister's house.
- Inform your partner that you are leaving, where you're going (if you haven't agreed beforehand), and when you are going to return. Even when you've very upset, you can say through gritted teeth, "I can't talk about this right now, I'll talk after I walk." Or, "I'm just going to Wal-Mart and I'll be back in an hour."

Be productive during your time-outs. Allow yourself to really cool off and calm down, but also examine your situation. If you're like some people, you'll spend at least the first half of your time thinking about everything your partner did wrong and why everything is his or her fault. When you're mad, it is really hard thinking about anything you did wrong, because you feel wronged. Try to find ways that help you blow off steam, let go of your anger, and help you see past your anger. Interestingly, it used to be thought that working on expressing your anger, verbally or physically, helped you get rid of your anger. Newer research has shown that focusing on your anger can actually make you even angrier or perpetuate anger. While it may be good, at first, to talk about your anger or do something physical to blow off steam, eventually thinking about other things or even other ways to see a problem will help you feel less angry and cool off quicker (see below).

4. DO FINISH A FIGHT

A huge mistake many couples make is to stop an argument, then never get back to it. Too many people just wake up the next day and act as if nothing happened. While this makes everyone feel good in the short-run, problems swept under the rug become the mess that people trip on later. It is important to finish the fight as soon as you can. Since most fights are over misunderstandings, if you would only talk, you will often find out that you did not intend to hurt each other.

It is okay to go to bed angry. Usually, you wake up in the morning and realize how silly the fight was, so it is easier to resolve the next day. Late night fights, when everyone is tired and cranky (or intoxicated) can be impossible times to solve real or imagined problems. On the other hand, when people get into a fight, it can cause deep distress that makes it impossible to sleep, because you're so angry or even worried that your relationship will be over! If you have to, miss a few hours of sleep to try to work out a problem.

TEN MINUTE TIP: COOLING OFF

- Physically release your anger through exercise. I go swimming and imagine punching the water or waves with my fists as I take a stroke. Some people run, some box, some walk, some go to the gym.
- Mentally release your anger. Try writing or journaling. Write out all your feelings and thoughts about the event. Writing helps you get your feelings out of your mind. Instead of recycling the same ideas, after you put some down on paper, your mind is free to think of different things, sometimes more things you are angry about, but eventually you might start writing down possible solutions.
- Verbally release your anger. Yell in a safe place, like a car, under water, or into a pillow. Talk to yourself or talk to a trusted friend on the phone—but not your partner's arch enemy (even in the family). You don't have to talk about the problem; sometimes any talk will distract you from your problems and let you think of other things.
- Clean your home. Cleaning will physically release your anger, but it can also clear your space of clutter, mentally and physically.
- Sleep. Fights are more likely to happen when people are tired. Rest first.
- Meditate or pray. Seek spiritual strength.
- Distract yourself from your anger. Listen to music, watch a funny movie, and listen to the talk radio.
- Go outside. Small spaces breed aggression. Clear your mind and body outdoors. Sit outside or walk. Breathe fresh air. Immerse yourself in nature and appreciate its beauty. Watch the moon and stars at night.
- Think hopeful thoughts. Try to remember a big fight in the past and remind yourself that you have overcome worse things.
- Become empathetic. Begin to think about the other person's point of view, not just your own.
- Have an attitude of gratitude. Try to remember aspects or memories of your relationship for which you feel grateful.

Sometimes, if you can't resolve everything, try to reassure each other that you'll talk the next day, even if you don't feel it at the time (because you are so angry that you secretly wonder if you'll be around tomorrow). Again, try to remember that you've had many fights, yet you're still together. After a fight, if you can't talk immediately or first thing in the morning, and one or both of you have to work that day, reassure each other that you will talk about it soon and work it out. Remember your love for and commitment to each other; remember that you both have to focus on your day and say, even if you are still upset, "Hey, we'll talk it out, okay? I love you!" Then, at your first opportunity, call each other on the phone, or if it's too big to be discussed during the work-day, agree to sit down and talk as soon as you get home, even if it will be late. It is very important to get back to each other as soon as possible to resolve conflicts, which create short-term anxieties, fears, and tensions. So often, minor conflicts grow into major conflicts when they are left unresolved.

5. NO SILENT VIOLENCE

Silent violence is when one person shuts down and refuses to talk about the conflict, sometimes for hours, sometimes by refusing to answer phone calls, sometimes by leaving and not returning, and sometimes for days. Silent violence is one of the worst dirty fighting techniques; it is a hostile form of avoidance and control. Silent violence is a form of emotional abuse, which causes a great deal of anxiety for the intended victim by creating hostility through silence. While some people stay silent because they are too mad or afraid to say the wrong thing, or they are avoiding the pain of an argument, a much better solution is to agree on the length of a time-out or cooling off period. A time-out is a part of a resolution strategy; silent violence is a form of passive-aggression and non-verbal emotional abuse.

People who have been on the receiving end of silent violence often feel a great deal of anxiety. They have no idea what their partners are angry about, since they aren't talking. When someone won't talk to them, they imagine all sorts of horrible things. People get very worried that their relationships or marriages are over. People wonder if the problem is too big to talk about and whether or not they'll be able to resolve the conflict. Sometimes people get physically ill with worry and anxiety after a long period of silence. At times, people break and decide to end the relationship themselves, to break the silence by leaving, rather than feel the pain of silent violence. Silent violence can destroy a relationship or marriage.

6. Do not fight to win

Fighting to win is street fighting, and it has no place in relationships. Fighting to win sounds like, "I'm right and you're wrong." Fighting to resolve conflict sounds like, "I can understand how you think and feel as you do, can you understand what I am saying?" Earlier in the chapter, you read about how fighting to win creates an illusion of control that can destroy your intimacy. Learn to communicate, not control, by listening and talking to each other. Let everybody say their whole side of the story without interruption. Their WHOLE side! Many fights are really misunderstandings in communication; one person thought that what the other person said or did was inconsiderate or intolerable, but the other person may not have said it or didn't mean it that way. Listen to the full story, and practice keeping your mouth shut while you're listening. In a fight, everyone wants to be right and everyone believes they are right, to a certain extent. Try, try, try to see how your partner might be a little right and acknowledge their "right points." Just doing this a little can change an entire fight, because you stopped fighting to win.

One of the really hard parts of relationships is being able to tolerate those difficult moments when you feel criticized, ignored, or hurt, sometimes for the wrong reasons, and to endure pain, anger, and suffering on bad days. But what makes a relationship last is a couple who's willing to fight fair and resolve conflicts that involve both partners' faults. If you can admit those faults, you can begin to really change yourself and your relationship, and being right or wrong in the past won't matter.

TEN MINUTE TIP: DO NOT PLAY THE DIVORCE CARD

This is a little aside about the divorce card. I'm going to tell you a little marital secret. Every couple, almost every individual (married or in a committed relationship), probably everyone reading this book, has been in a state of anger and thought something like, "I wish I'd never gotten married! If this continues, I want a divorce. Why did I ever marry him? If he doesn't change, I can't live like this anymore. If this is really what he thinks about me, I hate him! I want a divorce." It is really okay and normal to think this in the heat of anger, but learn to keep your mouth closed and keep your thoughts to yourselves, because 99.99 percent of the time you will find that those feelings will pass. Do not speak it and do not use the threat of a divorce. The only time that you use the divorce card is when it really needs to be played. Let me remind you: if it needs to be played, don't play it when you're really, really mad and/or drunk and/or horny, late at night. If the divorce card really needs to be played, it will be just as effective 24 hours later—because divorce is forever. Once you have played it, you can't take it back. So just hold on to that card and don't say your feelings out loud because you'll probably regret it the next day. If you really want a divorce, you will still feel that way when you are calm and cooled off.

If you are in a nonmarried relationship, compare the divorce card to a threat to move out or kick someone out, in the heat of the moment. This threat is a power play used when fighting to win. The only time that people use the divorce card over and over again is when they're trying to say, "Shut up. I want the fight over," or when they are using it to really hurt and reject someone. Most people are not serious about wanting a relationship to end; they are fighting to win by using fear and intimidation. It is a very powerful dirty fighting technique, because it can scare someone into doing whatever you want them to do. But beware: Using the divorce card or other relationship threats repeatedly can backfire. Eventually people get tired of being threatened, and sometimes they'll take you up on it in a state of anger, and move out of your life forever. If you're just overreacting when you're angry, as many people do, and simply thinking these relationship ending thoughts, stop talking and ask to take a time-out, which is what you really need.

7. ADMIT WHEN YOU ARE WRONG

No fight can be resolved unless each person can admit their faults or "growth areas." A relationship that works must include being able to admit when you are wrong! Everyone wants to be right, but problems cannot be resolved until each person is able to admit when he or she made a mistake. Almost always, when your partner is telling you something bad about yourself, there is at least a little portion of truth in what is said. Don't ignore this valuable information, as painful as it is to hear. Look for the grain of truth…like the grain of sand that irritates the oyster enough to develop a pearl…of wisdom. Many people who have been divorced later realize that there was some truth in what their first spouse told them about their faults.

> **You have to stop yelling or telling people what they are doing wrong, and start by admitting your own faults. Admitting you're wrong stops a fight and starts a discussion.**

TEN MINUTE TIP: THE NAKED MIRROR OF RELATIONSHIPS

Okay, this is the hard part, but this is how you really resolve problems. Each of you must look into the naked mirror of relationships. I'm not telling you to put the other person's face in front of that mirror. I'm telling you to look at yourself in the mirror. You need to think, while looking in the naked mirror of relationships, about what the person was screaming at you or telling you that you did wrong when you were fighting. You know it's true: Sometimes your partner is right and you did something wrong. Work hard to find the grain of truth or the percentage of ownership of your fault in the problem. It may be that the conflict is only 10 percent your problem or even 1 percent of the problem. But there is usually a grain of truth in what the person has to say in anger. Don't ignore this valuable information, as painful as it may be to hear. Many, many people who get divorced later realize, "Yeah my first husband was right, even if it's to a small extent, and I really should have listened to him when he said [fill in the blank]."

You must look in the mirror and you must find that grain of truth, and then you must admit when you're wrong. Even if it is 99 percent your partner's fault, how you really resolve problems is that you BOTH take responsibility for your tiny, tiny incidental part of the problem.

Later, look at the section below on self-examination to help you identify your shortcomings, faults, and growth areas—where you can improve—without having to be told about them in a fight.

8. LEARN TO SAY "I'M SORRY"

A relationship that works includes being able to admit that you're wrong *and* saying you're sorry. My mother—a mother of 10 children and married for over 50 years now—once said that one of the most important needs for people, after eating and sex, is to "be right" (and she's right about that!). Everyone wants to be right, at least some of the time, but problems cannot be resolved until each person is able to admit when they made a mistake, and then say, "I'm sorry." Learn to say you're sorry even if the problem is not all your fault.

Besides saying you're sorry, you need to take turns with who apologizes first. Look closely at yourself in your relationship. Are you as likely to be the one to approach your partner and say you were wrong? Or are you still fighting to win, meaning you are never wrong, and your partner always has to approach you, admitting his or her faults and most of the blame, before you admit you're wrong, if you do?

> **You have to be the one to say you're sorry *first*...
> at least some of the time.**

THE FIETSAM APOLOGY

I already said to admit you're wrong and say you're sorry, but this is a little qualification on that. Be able to say you're sorry without a comma and a "BUT" after it. Now, I'm going to tell you a little story about the Fietsam apology. Give me just a second here. This one's hard. I had to look in the mirror for a moment first. I have eight brothers and sisters, and we were all at a family Christmas with all the in-laws, all eight spouses, sitting around the big kitchen table, talking loudly, while our 30 children ran around us. My brother, Chad, ran into the kitchen to bring a diaper bag from the car for his wife, Chris. The diaper bag errand took an extended period of time, and he was supposed to be getting baby food as well. His wife had gotten desperate, listening to a screaming starving toddler, and mashed up a banana to feed the baby by the time he got back. As sweet as she normally is, she glared at him when he walked in the room and said in a hushed one, though gritted teeth, "Where were you?" Chad looked back at her and said, "I'm sorry it took me so long, but if you hadn't put the diaper bag way underneath the back seat where I couldn't find it, then we wouldn't have had such a problem." In truth, he had been dawdling, talking to a family member before he went out to go get the bag. My husband commented, where everybody could hear him and said, "Oh, well that was a great Fietsam apology." The in-laws all perked up their ears. "What's a Fietsam apology?" My husband—Jack, who obviously didn't want to have sex for the rest of the holiday season retorted—"Oh, that's when you say 'I'm sorry, but it's your fault.'" Of course, the in-laws all laughed loudly. Too loudly.

Fietsam is, of course, my maiden name.

Jack, apparently, not planning on having sex until Valentine's Day, continued, "Yeah, you know, the Fietsam apology is when you say, 'I'm sorry, but if you weren't so sensitive, then there wouldn't be a problem.' Or 'I'm sorry, but if you didn't do this, then I wouldn't have done that, so it's really your fault.'" And, of course, the in-laws got a big kick out of that, too. They all had a huge laugh about that for a few hours. But I learned a lesson: that my husband was right and I actually did do that when I apologized! When I said I was sorry, I almost always used an excuse and turned it back on him, basically saying, "Well, I'm sorry, Jack, but you if you hadn't [fill in the blank]—so it's your fault" or excusing my rudeness I'd say, "Well, I'm sorry, but I'm just being honest and you're too sensitive."

It isn't an apology and it isn't admitting you're wrong when you say, "I'm sorry, BUT." You have to cut off the excuses, and simply admit your fault. Until you can each admit your fault, you will continue arguing, trying to get your partner to admit his part of the problem, even when part of the problem is yours. You may try and try and try to keep arguing until your partner admits he is wrong first, but if you want to stop the arguing, grow up and start by looking in the naked mirror of marriage at yourself first.

9. SOLVE THE REAL PROBLEM

Couples escalate problems from minor problems to discussions of someone's personality issues to questioning break up or divorce!

Keep focused on the problem that you were originally fighting over. If you're talking about who left dishes in the sink, stick to the dishes: Don't jump to calling him or her a slob and a lousy partner. It's the dishes. Yet, most of the time people start big fights over little things that just get out of hand. So stick to the problem, when it's a little problem, and don't let it escalate to the point that you are thinking about ending the relationship.

Sometimes there really are big things that need to be discussed: These are real problems. Real problems include differences of opinion over money, sex, children, friends, family, time spent together, and lifestyle, such as socializing and where or when to buy or fix up a home. Some problems are not solved overnight or sometimes even over the course of an entire marriage, and we'll talk about how to work on solving these more difficult problems next. For now, work on solving minor problems by talking about the issue directly, addressing each other's needs and wants, and negotiating. Here's a guide.

TEN MINUTE TIP: BRAINSTORM REAL SOLUTIONS FOR REAL PROBLEMS

Brainstorm together, with a pad of paper and pencil. Write down all of your ideas on how to solve the problem, from the obvious to the absurd. For example, let's say you've had a fight with your boss. The solutions might include:

Quit your job, tell her off, go to her boss, pretend it didn't happen, listen to her side, call in sick, bring a coworker in with you for a meeting, call the human resources department, send your husband/wife in to talk to them, change your career.

Throw out all of your wild ideas, then sort through the rest together. Laugh and be loving, then work toward solving the problem by using compromise or taking turns to decide on which solution to use.

10. TAKE TURNS BEING RIGHT

Try compromising. Compromise alone can solve many problems.

For some problems, giving in and taking less is more in the long-run. Unfortunately, sometimes compromise is highly overrated when one person is adamant about what they want. At times, compromise can make you feel like you can't get what you really want, which is one reason people keep fighting, repeating their argument over and over again until they are "heard." You can't compromise on going to Disneyworld when Disneyworld's where you want to go! You can't go halfway to Disneyworld, stop in Kansas, and be satisfied. Instead, do what you learned in kindergarten.

Try taking turns. When you take turns, eventually everyone can take a turn being right, getting their own way, and getting more of what they want! For example, you take turns by going to Disneyworld one year, and then going to the NASCAR races the next, if that's what each of you wants. You can take turns with who gets a new car, who cleans the bathtub, how you spend the money or how you get rid of debt, or even how to solve the problem of disciplining children. When you take turns, you show each other that you care, that you matter to each other, and it translates into feeling good about each other and improving intimacy, because you are a loving team!

TAKING TURNS RAISING KIDS

Taking turns works great when deciding how to solve a problem with kids because there is usually no single right approach; it is trial and error for what works with each child. Yet we all know problems with kids can put a wedge between parents. And then you're mad at each other and you don't have sex, right?

Let's say you've got a problem with getting homework done. First, admit that you've both got a problem helping this child to get homework done. You can't play the blame game, with one parent trying to solve the problem by trying one thing and the other person looking on and saying, "Oh, you're not doing it right!" Okay, Mr. Big Mouth,

Ms. Perfectly-Right-All-The-Time: You try it. You try to solve the problem.

Let the other parent take a turn and try to figure it out so that each parent gets an opportunity to try out their ideas while the other parent watches and learns. In reality, either parent may learn their partner was right and can support them and/or they may learn something new. Or you might find out that both of you are wrong, so you can join in feeling helpless, and then work together to brainstorm new solutions. Try to remember: There is often no single right answer. Give each other a chance to try out different solutions.

Avoid the Blame Game

Another variation of the blame game is when partners blame the other person all the time, yet they aren't willing to come up with suggestions or make decisions. When a decision is finally made and it turns out poorly, the decision-maker is blamed. Take warning: If someone isn't willing to be a part of the solution, then that partner has no right to blame someone else for solving the problem, even if it was wrong. It is cowardly to not make any decisions, then turn around and blame someone for making the wrong ones. If people can't stand up for what they believe in and take their turn being right when the decision is being made, they have no right to criticize. The decision-maker shouldn't take criticism either, when he or she had the courage to try and solve a problem! As the old saying goes, "You're either a part of the solution, or a part of the problem."

Resentments

> Unresolved conflicts create resentment. Resentment turns into contempt. Contempt is the foundation upon which divorce is built.

Now that you've learned to fight right, you should be able to resolve any conflict, right? Much resentment comes from conflicts that cou-

129

ples simply can't seem to resolve. Often, these conflicts are from either a lack of agreement about matters or breaking agreements that have been made. Many couples fight the same fights over and over again, trying to get their partners to do what they said they were going to do or to change their mind about what they won't agree to do.

What's Your Agreement?

What's your agreement about money? Sex? Kids? Housework? Vacations?

Every person has negotiable and nonnegotiable wishes, desires, and demands within a relationship. Nonnegotiable matters may be about fidelity, drug or alcohol use, use of pornography, or even smaller personal matters; these matters are not up for agreement, and they are individual requirements in their relationship. For example, when I married my husband, he agreed to travel to Michigan to visit with my family every Christmas. I had moved away from my family to South Carolina to be with Jack. He agreed that every Christmas, we would go to my large family's Christmas reunion, and we have every year. It is nonnegotiable, but he also agreed on it. If he did not keep his promise, I would be very resentful. When nonnegotiable agreements are broken, so is trust in a relationship, and resentments develop. When promises are kept, appreciation is cultivated, as is respect, admiration, and gratitude.

Negotiable matters can vary widely among individuals and couples. These may concern the way in which household duties are divided, finances are arranged, children are cared for, family gatherings are attended, or how much time couples spend together. In new relationships, individuals bring expectations about what they think they should agree to. During the dating years, many of these matters are discussed, values are shared, and some expectations are outlined and agreed upon. No couple can talk about all of the relationship expectations prior to making a commitment to each other or marriage, which is why people are still fighting in marriages after 50 years! Each set of changing responsibilities, duties, and activities within a household and a couple's relationship needs to be discussed and agreed upon so that expectations can be understood, agreements made, and obligations met in daily life.

Too often in relationships, people NEVER make these agreements, and when their expectations aren't met, they are unhappy or have a fight. Some people neglect to make BASIC agreements, like about monogamy, and they are surprised and betrayed when someone cheats, while their partners act blameless because they "didn't understand" or have an agreement.

> **All couples have to make agreements on important matters, or they will fight.**

Ask yourself: Do you have agreements or merely assumptions about the way you want things in your life? Do you have "normal expectations?" Do you meet "normal expectations?" When people don't agree on fulfilling what their partner assumes are normal expectations, they will have resentments. And they will be less likely to care about meeting your normal expectations, such as having an active sex life. Couples with conflicts either don't make agreements about important matters, don't agree on expectations, or break agreements, which is how resentments are created.

EXPECTATIONS

Resentments arise from people either breaking agreements or refusing to make agreements on matters of importance. As a therapist, it is amazing to see the incredibly wide variety of relationship expectations and agreements. It is also interesting to see what people fight about, and to find out what matters to them.

People are different. They are going to disagree. They will not always agree to disagree. The question is: Is a disagreement reasonable? Are people being fair with each other? Is one person being selfish? Are both people carrying their share of responsibilities? These types of disputes often land on a therapist's couch. For example, in childrearing, it is often the mother who will get up in the middle of the night to feed a new-born infant. Is it a reasonable expectation that the father/partner takes a turn getting up, losing sleep, for a nonbreastfeeding child? Or is that the mother's responsibility? Usually a mother gets up for midnight feedings, while the father sleeps, sometimes because he's working and she's not in the beginning. So when she returns to work or school, should the fathers do all the feedings, half of them, or any of them? If the mother's expectation is that the father should help and do half the feedings, but he will not agree to do any, she will be resentful. What is fair? What is right? Why didn't they talk about this before they had a baby? Often, couples have conflicts over making these agreements. A therapist can help couples agree on making agreements, as a mediator, to resolve these types of conflicts.

UNMET EXPECTATIONS

What if the new father agreed to do half of the midnight feedings, but he doesn't get out of bed when the baby cries, and the mother has to do it? An expectation is unmet, and there is resentment.

If you make an agreement and you then break it, your partner will resent you. Resentment kills intimacy and sex lives. Loving feelings and a sexual relationship can die over resentments and unmet expectations, along with passion. So you have to ask yourself, are you meeting your partner's expectations in a reasonable way or is resentment affecting your intimacy?

SELF-EXAMINATION: YOUR LOOK IN THE MIRROR

Before you head for a couples therapist, a sex therapist, or a divorce lawyer, try a serious self-examination. You need to ask yourself hard questions and be painfully honest with yourself while looking in the naked mirror of relationships. Be responsible for your actions (or inaction). Don't wait until things are critical in your relationship or wait to say at the last minute, "I'll do ANYTHING to keep our relationship together." Do anything NOW.

TEN MINUTE TIP: TAKE RESPONSIBILITY IN YOUR RELATIONSHIP

- Don't wait until you're single to do your share of housework.
- Don't wait until you're single to get into shape emotionally or physically.
- Don't wait until you're single to do your share as a parent.
- Don't wait until you're single to establish your job/career.
- Don't take advantage of a relationship or marriage to be complacent about yourself.

ASK YOURSELF THIS QUESTION: WOULD I WANT TO BE MARRIED TO ME?

Would you want a relationship with you? With your personality, your ability to love and to give love, your ability to make love and have ravishing sex, your ability to be a friend, your ability to listen, to be there for someone in the ups and downs and trials of life, to coparent with, to share a bed with at night, to share a tube of toothpaste or to live with day to day, would you want to share a life with you?

Ask yourself this: Do you do the things to take care of yourself that you used to when you were single, or do you leave it up to your partner? In fact, if you were suddenly single, what *would* you be doing or taking care of that your partner handles, simply by default? These things might be your laundry, including picking up the dry cleaning, planning for and preparing meals, picking up around the house, spending one-on-one time with the kids, paying bills, buying gifts for your family, walking the dog, planning vacations, doing car maintenance, or finding a babysitter. Think about these day-to-day

Self-Examination

Your personality

Am I an interesting person?

Am I patient?

Am I in decent physical shape?

Am I sexy?

Am I fun?

Am I loving and nurturing?

Am I too demanding of myself or others?

Am I obsessive/compulsive?

Am I spontaneous and energetic?

Am I a slob or excessively neat?

Am I a good conversationalist?

Am I a happy, positive person or am I depressed and negative?

Am I a good listener?

Am I good company?

Am I the person I want to be?

Look for addictions:

Do I spend too much?

Do I take too many risks or gamble?

Am I having an affair, even in cyberspace?

Do I work too much?

Do I drink too much?

Do I abuse drugs?

Am I very overweight?

Do I smoke?

Do I endanger my health or scare my partner with any of my life habits?

Am I the person I want to be?

Am I the person I promised I would be?

Will my partner be a better person for having known me?

tasks that are the normal details of life. If you aren't doing them, who is? These are the types of tasks partners expect you to do that when, left unmet, cause a wedge in your relationships.

Conversely, what do you do to contribute to your relationship that makes your partner's life better? Ask your partner what kind of things they resent. Ask how you can help to change those feelings of resentment. You may also have resentments that need to be addressed. Most partners want to please each other, but they can't read each other's mind when it comes to the little things in life that can bring joy. Together, you can help each other examine your lives and your expectations, and uncover your unmet expectations and resentments. You must be willing to listen, but also be reasonable with yourself and your partner. If you cannot agree on what are reasonable expectations and meet them, you can consult friends, family, or a couples and sex therapist.

ANGER CAN KILL SEXUAL DESIRE

Problems solving conflicts lead to arguments, which lead to resentments. Resentments make love and sexual feelings fade. Sometimes there are differences of sexual values, opinions, desires, and behaviors that develop into long-standing disagreements. Couples learn to avoid certain subjects to keep the peace, and they learn to live with differences of opinions on some subjects, too. However, avoiding serious issues, such as a sexual problem, causes relationship problems. Left unresolved, these impasses create distance between people. Sometimes that distance is two bedrooms away or two months between sexual liaisons. Differences must be worked out or they'll work many couples out of a relationship, sexual or otherwise. What really makes a relationship work is having the courage to fight right, so you can enjoy the intimacy of friendship, companionship, affection, and sex, and the trust that your love will be there with you, throughout your life.

CHAPTER

7

Maintenance Sex for Busy Couples

Maintenance sex builds on the foundation of sexual communication and intimacy unique to monogamy, marriage, and long-lasting, loving relationships. Maintenance sex is an essential component of the Ten Minute Sexual Solution that goes beyond intimacy and deals directly with meeting sexual needs within a relationship and within a culture that puts sexual needs last. Maintenance sex is 10 minutes of sexual play to meet one or both partners' sexual needs in a brief but pleasurable moment of time. Sharing maintenance sex is one of the ways couples can manage having different sexual desires and needs. Learning as a couple to handle sexual differences is an important part of a loving relationship. Communicating about sexual expectations and addressing these sexual differences is a caring way to share love and sexual satisfaction in a long-term relationship or marriage. You can change your entire sexual mapping by embracing maintenance sex to create sexual synchronicity.

CREATING SEXUAL SYNCHRONICITY

The most common sexual problem couples encounter is discrepant or different sexual desires. Discrepant sexual desire is clinically defined as when a couple has different sexual desires and one person in the relationship is chronically and greatly distressed over their sexual frequency. Obviously, this broad definition can include almost all couples at one time or another over the duration of a long-term relationship or marriage. Nearly 60 percent of all married couples and 44 percent of non-married couples have sex less than once a week[1]. Coincidently, 50 percent of all couples report having sex two-four or more times per week, while 50 percent of couples report "differences in sexual desire." It is likely that couples who have sex more than twice a week are sexually in sync, and the other half of couples aren't. Some individuals have a desire for sex every day, while some individuals prefer having sex once a month or less, simply because this is "normal" for them. Unfortunately, if these two people are married or committed to each other, they will definitely have a problem with discrepant sexual desire!

> **The bottom line is that approximately 50 percent of all couples need a solution to create sexual synchronicity in their relationship or marriage.**

Chapter 2 described the sexual struggles couple often experience when they have sexual differences. While it is normal for couples to have sexual differences or differences in sexual desires, it is destructive to have sexual power struggles that damage emotional intimacy, loving feelings, and trust. There are several ways that couples can handle these sexual differences that are not destructive. Couples with sexual desire discrepancies or substantial sexual changes that alter sexual expression, such as medical problems, can choose to create a "new normal." A new normal can mean a very new definition of sexual expression in order to share love and physically pleasure each other to create sexual synchronicity, including maintenance sex, a new way to share affection and increase your sexual frequency.

What is Maintenance Sex?

Maintenance sex is part of the Ten Minute Sexual Solution that will help you get in sync sexually. Maintenance sex is giving each other 10 minutes to spend uninterrupted time alone for physically loving one another. Maintenance sex is a special way for busy couples to share sexuality. Once a couple has taken the time to create a foundation of sexual communication, emotional intimacy, and trust, they can create flexibility in the way they define and express their sexualities together. Maintenance sex can include a variety of sexual acts, including sex with your hands, oral sex, and sexual intercourse, for one or both partners. Maintenance sex is a way to maintain your sexual relationship with brief interludes of sexual play. Many people feel they simply don't have time for sex, but most don't realize the biological reality of how long sex lasts, depending on your *sexual mapping* (see page 140).

THE BIOLOGICAL TRUTH ABOUT SEX

The truth will set you free: The average man takes two minutes to get excited enough to have sex. The average woman takes eight minutes to get aroused for sex. The average human coitus is just two minutes long: from thrust to finish. If you take eight minutes to fool around long enough to get everyone turned on and two minutes to have sex: Voilá! You have a part of *The Ten Minute Sexual Solution:* Maintenance sex for busy couples!

Maintenance sex is taking advantage of our biological reality, and taking a little time for each other to meet each other's basic sexual needs. Maintenance sex can create quality quickies for caring couples. Maintenance sex can include simply having sexual play for one partner with oral sex, "having a handie" (manually stimulating someone with your hand), or just a little bit of sexual intercourse. Maintenance sex can include limited foreplay, but enough kissing and caressing to get excited and physiologically sexually aroused to enjoy a few minutes of sexual intercourse. It might include many types of sexual touch and sexual play, just enough for one or both partners to have sexual pleasure or reach a climax, too. It includes ravishing each other, out of want and love. Maintenance sex includes times when only one person is interested, and the other person isn't. It can be helpful when you have different timing or levels of sexual desire, to fill in the gaps between passionate lovemaking. It can be a quickie for both people to have sexual climaxes, or neither, depending on who wants what, when.

> **Maintenance sex is about being accommodating to your partner's sexual needs, even if you don't really have any at the moment…out of love.**

Important: I am not talking about someone NOT wanting sex, but sometimes one person may not really be "in the mood." Sometimes the uninterested partner can have a really good time, too, when they weren't even thinking about wanting sex! As you will learn in chapter 8, sexual desire can be rekindled with sexual touch, rather than waiting for desire to happen spontaneously. Maintenance sex builds sexual trust and love, knowing you are there for each other. Please remember that your partner is there for you, and you are there for your partner. This is about being friends and lovers.

Most couples have never thought of having brief interludes of playful sex, outside the context of a full course of lovemaking. Some people have quickies, but that is often limited to quick sexual intercourse. While maintenance sex can and does include sexual intercourse, it can also NOT include any sexual intercourse. Or it might include sexual intercourse for a couple of minutes, but not for a long time, or not for the purpose of both people having an orgasm.

One or neither partner may have an orgasm during maintenance sex. Some people might ask, "So what's the purpose of having maintenance sex, if you're not going to have an orgasm?" First of all, not everyone seeks or wants to have an orgasm during a brief interlude of sexual play. Second, being sexually playful is not always for the purpose of a sexual release. On the other hand, some people, especially women, might have two or three orgasms in 10 minutes, from oral sex, hand stimulation, or a vibrator. The point is that people can be sexually inventive, creative, and playful, having quick sexual moments that they do not ordinarily think of sharing, when the demands for orgasms or a certain sexual structure are no longer made, if you change your sexual mapping.

SEXUAL MAPPING

Sexual mapping is a phrase for what you do sexually, when you have sex. Often, couples share a similar sexual map or sexual routine when they share lovemaking. Basically, this means that couples tend to repeat the same sexual behaviors with each other, over time. A sexual map may include the way sex is started or initiated, and what couples do for foreplay, during sex, and after sex. Changing your sexual mapping is a way to create a new sexual script.

A SAMPLE SEXUAL MAP: ASHLEY AND RYAN

Ashley asks Ryan to go to bed. Ryan knows that if Ashley asks him to bed, then she wants to have sex. He knows she likes to take a shower first and wants him to take a shower before they have sex, so he goes upstairs to take a shower, without saying anything, a few minutes after Ashley already went upstairs. Ryan gets upstairs shortly after Ashley gets out of the shower. They pass in the bathroom, smile at each other, and Ryan showers without saying a word. Ryan meets Ashley in bed, naked. He lights the candle next to their bed. He reaches over and slowly undresses her, removing the sexy nightie she wore for him. He lies behind her and begins to rub her shoulders. While her shoulders are being rubbed, she presses her buttocks up against his erection. When she is ready, she turns around and kisses him. When he is ready to stop kissing, he touches her breasts. She reaches down and strokes his penis. Now, he knows it is okay to touch her genitals. He strokes her clitoris until she has an orgasm. After she has an orgasm, he gets on top of her, and they have intercourse. She never has an orgasm during sex, so when Ryan is finished, sex is over. They lie together, usually with her head on his chest. They may talk for a few minutes, and then they go to sleep.

YOUR SEXUAL MAP

Couples have their own sexual signatures and sexual mapping. Sometimes they have slight variations on their sexual mapping, but couples often develop sexual mapping that is very similar, and is repeated over time. If the mapping changes, it is often the same two or three changes, such as adding oral sex or one or two different sexual positions. Usually, each partner has the same number of orgasms each time they have sex: one for him, one for her, or two for her, one for her or two for him, or one for him, and so on.

Thinking about sex this way, do you see a pattern in your sexual mapping? How do you prepare for sex? How do you each initiate sex? Who initiates sex? How much kissing do you do? Do you use lube and who gets it out and when is it applied? Who comes first? Who comes last? What do you do when you're finished? Couples often develop one, two, or three (but often one) single sexual map that is used consistently over and over again. Most of the time similar sexual mapping is used because a couple has found that these are the sexual behaviors that work for them, consistently bring them sexual pleasure, or have been discussed to be safe or "allowed," in some cases. Most often, couples simply get into a habit of a sexual map because it consistently brings them both sexual pleasure and a sexual release that is satisfying.

Over time, partners tend to talk less and less about their mapping, having discussed long ago what they like or dislike sexually, and doing what works for them the best. Some couples get into sexual routines that may change every few years or so, but when they have a routine that is working, they'll stick to it for a while.

While some couples are perfectly happy with their current sexual mapping, some couples are bored, some individuals are less than satisfied, and others are quite dissatisfied. In some cases, running through the entire sexual map every time you share a sexual interlude can take a long time! Going through *all* the sexual motions you go through or having *all* the sexual behaviors every single time can create sexual routines that take over an hour. While some people are happy with this, others find that sex takes too long, takes too much preparation, and becomes sexual drudgery in some cases. For some people, when they think about having sex and going through their entire sexual routine or sexual map, they want to avoid sex because it simply takes too much time and energy.

Changing Your Sexual Map

One of the incredible advantages of the Ten Minute Sexual Solution is that you have a new opportunity to change your sexual mapping! You can use some of the skills you learned, such as rating your sexual desire, using your sexual language, and practicing communication to tell each other what you want and do not want sexually. But one of the most exciting parts of the Ten Minute Sexual Solution is that you can change your sexual mapping and share just one part or many parts of your favorite sexual menu for having maintenance sex! You can create new sexual scripts or have experiences that don't use your old sexual map at all! Maintenance sex can allow you to have exciting, interesting, and titillating sexual surprises that can completely change your sex life!

All you need to do is give each other permission, and sometimes encouragement, to have maintenance sex become a part of your sexual mapping. Often, couples need permission to ask and receive simple changes in their sexual routine. If you can agree on having maintenance sex, or agree on changing your sexual map, to allow for only 10 minutes of sexual sharing, you can begin to have many miniature sexual interludes, when one of you in your relationship is not really in the mood or up to sharing your entire sexual routine together. While this may sound silly or too simple to do, this concept of giving each other permission to have maintenance sex, not EVERYTHING sex, can amazingly change the entire map of your sexual relationship! Of course, you have to have a foundation of trust, emotional intimacy, and—most importantly—communication, but with those components of the Ten Minute Sexual Solution in place, you can completely change and excite your sexual relationship!

Here's a sample: When was the last time you jumped on top of your partner on the couch of your living room, not violently, but passionately hugging and pushing him or her down on the couch, giving a wet, long kiss? Or maybe to press against their body against yours? With no strings attached that it had to lead to sex? Or asking to give or receive oral sex, for just a couple of minutes, not necessarily to orgasm, but just for sexual play?

If you asked most people, they would enjoy parts of that sexual sampling if it didn't involve a demand for sex, or a demand for their having an orgasm, or a demand for having an entire sexual scenario—but ONLY if, when they said no, stop, or go, it would be okay! Some people are afraid to kiss or be seductive or sexually playful because then it would mean they would have to or need to complete their entire sexual journey or map. And no one's "in the mood" for all of that all the time! But most people are in the mood for being sexually playful much more often! All it takes is permission, communication, and embracing maintenance sex as a part of your sexual relationship.

DEALING WITH SEXUAL FRUSTRATION

So many times, with everyone's jammed schedules, our physical desires are not in sync. But sometimes one person is...really desperate. This is where maintenance sex really works for busy couples. For any couple who has different or discrepant sexual desires, maintenance sex can bridge the sexual gap, the distance that creates a sexual wedge between you. When one person wants more sex, it is sexually frustrating for BOTH people. A lot of men and a lot of women, too, are in relationships and marriages where they are feeling sexually frustrated! More and more women have stronger sex drives than their husbands and they want to simply, frankly, have more sex! If this is you, then maintenance sex is a great solution to solve the problem, when you love each other and you want to stay together, stay faithful, and stay true to your marital vows of being the only sexual partners for each other!

A lot of women ask, "So what am I going to get out of this? It takes me longer than 10 minutes to get something out of sex, if you know what I mean!"

Yes, I know what you mean. Some women know that it takes them longer than 10 minutes to think about sex, feel any desire for sex, or even get sexually aroused...and that doesn't count how long it takes to have an orgasm! Many women need a transition from life to thinking sexual thoughts, and 10 minutes isn't going to do it for them.

Part of the Ten Minute Sexual Solution is to increase the intimacy in your relationship with 10 minutes a day of loving talk and play. Most women feel a need to have emotional closeness prior to desiring sexual closeness. Increasing intimacy may allow you to have your emotional needs met and possibly increase your sexual desire, as well. This way, when it's time for maintenance sex, a woman may be better able to enjoy that 10 minutes!

If you are a woman who takes longer than 10 minutes to get aroused or have an orgasm, or if you are not orgasmic at all, you may be concerned about getting pleasure from maintenance sex. Many women suffer from the frustration of not being orgasmic or struggling with slow arousal and hard to reach climaxes, let alone desiring sex. Chapters 8 and 9 directly address women to help you break through mental sexual barriers, awaken your sexual self, and increase your sexual desire, as well as detailing how to become more easily orgasmic, whether you now have regular orgasms or none at all. Chapter 9 is aimed at helping you to focus on meeting your sexual needs, especially when life doesn't give you the time (or energy) to make sex worthwhile for you. Claim your own sexuality to it fullest potential, and you may find you will receive pleasure in 10 minute sexual interludes.

Some men wonder how they are going to "have sex," when they aren't in the mood. Due to the wisdom of the penis, many men can't just "will" an erection to appear on a moment's notice, when they're not interested in sex! But sex doesn't have to include an erection. Many women enjoy the pleasure of touch, the pleasure of hugging and kissing, and the pleasure of sexual stimulation from your fingers, hands, and oral sex.

If you are among the many, many people who are in a relationship with a partner that has a stronger sex drive than you, what can you do? Couples know some of the destructive ways they have handled differences in sexual desire in the past. Is it any wonder why people avoid sex, fake orgasms, or even hate sex? To manage sexual frustration, some people give in to sex that is unwanted, but it can backfire and make people hate sex more! A better solution is to deal directly with sexual differences and address the issue of expectations and sexual accommodation, including maintenance sex.

Sexual Differences in Monogamous Relationships

YOUR SEXUAL CYCLES

- How often do you like to have sex, either by yourself or with your partner?
- How often does your partner like to have sex, either by themselves or with you?
- How often do you feel like you really NEED to have sex, or you start feeling sexually frustrated or sexually desperate! Do you know?
- Does your partner know your sexual desires and needs? Have you talked about it?

It is essential to know and understand you and your partner's sex drive, or how often you feel the need to have sex with each other. It helps to understand and compare your sexual drives, how they vary from time to time and in different situations, and to determine your areas of compatibility and difference. For most couples, knowing your partner sexually just makes good sense when you have a monogamous relationship, excluding all other sexual partners. When you are married and/or monogamous partners, talking about your sexual drive and needs is important, so you can find out what each other needs and expects from your sexual relationship.

Sometimes couples simply don't talk about sex, and both partners have no idea what the other partner wants sexually. Sexual silence breeds resentments when people's expectations aren't met, even when they are simply sexual assumptions, because people have absolutely no way to meet their partner's needs or even their own!

Use your sexual communication skills from chapter 4, remember to be accepting, and talk about your sexual drive or sexual cycle. Your sexual cycle is how often you like to have sex, including sexual variations that can go in cycles or patterns in your life. For example, some women have more sexual drive before their period. Some men like to have sex a few days a week, but if they don't have sex for 10 days, they know they'll get very sexually frustrated and irritable. Work on understanding and accepting both of your individual sex drives for better or for worse. Since all individuals have different sexual needs at different times throughout a long-term relationship, communicating about your sexual drive over time is very important.

SEXERCISE #11

YOUR SEXUAL CYCLE

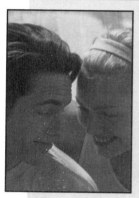

Discuss your own sexual cycle. Discuss how often you want or desire sex, as well as your feelings when you do not share sexual connections. Discuss how often you may be willing to share sex with your partner, even if it is just maintenance sex. Be realistic. As stated, some people say they would like to have sex every day, but even when it is available all the time, they don't always want it. Life and activities get in the way of sex at the end of the day, and men and women both get tired, even when sex is available. In thinking about these questions, be real about your answers. How often do you really want sex? How long between sexual interludes does it take before you get "horny" again? How long is your sexual cycle, meaning how long does it take before you really start getting sexually desirous or frustrated when you don't have sex? Take time to share who you are sexually, being compassionate and accepting with each other's honesty.

SEXPECTATIONS

Now that you've talked about who you are sexually, in terms of your sexual cycles, what are your "sexpectations"—sexual expectations? How often do you expect to share sex, given the differences in your sexual cycles? Do you expect each other to meet these sexpectations? More important than sexual frequency, what are your sexpectations when it comes to sexual pleasure? For some people, experiencing sexual pleasure is more important than how often they share sex. What kind of sexual mapping do you enjoy? How has it changed over time?

As with all other matters in your life, sex matters. Sexual matters need to be discussed, and you need to make sexual agreements. However, people disagree greatly how on to make these agreements, what are normal expectations for sex, and how much responsibility sexual partners have to meet these needs. Even therapists, who act as mediators for areas of conflict, cannot give you a set of "normal" sexpectations for couples because of your very individual feelings about sexuality. Other areas in your life that require agreement, such as money or housework or childrearing, do not involve the very personal feelings and individual variation, as well as emotional connection, as does sex. Yet in every area, each partner in a relationship takes a varying degree of responsibility for that area of life. Sex is the only area of life that must have a shared responsibility, since you have to do it together. People can make their own money, clean their own houses, raise their own kids, but they can't have partnered sex alone. So…

How much responsibility do partners have to each other when it comes to sexpectations?

What are "reasonable" sexpectations?

Unfortunately, most people don't talk about or make sexual agreements before they get married or committed, because they often assume their sexual relationship *will be the same or only slightly different than it was before marriage*! They assume that since they love each other and want each other all the time, the same feelings will always be there and never change. People do change. People's sexuality evolves over time. At least half of couples get to the point that their sexual desires are incompatible.

Nobody is *responsible* for meeting your, or your partner's, every sexual need, but how much responsibility are you willing to take for each other's sexpectations? What partners can do is to be caring lovers, whom desire to understand and meet sexpectations, while taking responsibility for their own sexuality, including maintaining their own healthy sexual identity. Most monogamous partners desire to please their lovers to varying extents. Some people seek to meet their partner's every sexual need. Sadly, other people couldn't care less about their partner's sexual needs and refuse to take any sexual responsibility in their relationship. As with other relationship responsibilities that go unmet, when sexpectations are unmet, conflicts will arise, and resentments can develop. Sexual resentments can lead to feelings of anger, dissatisfaction, or contempt, which can destroy a relationship. Seeking to meet sexpectations and create sexual compatibility is a loving act. Sex is a shared responsibility in a monogamous relationship.

> **Learn to manage the normal variations in sexpectations over a long-term relationship to share sexual trust and satisfaction.**

The first step in managing sexpectations is to let it be okay if someone wants more sex or less sex, rather than trying to change it. It's like trying to control someone's appetite for food: ridiculous and impossible! Second, adopting a loving attitude of wanting to please each other sexually, given that you are each other's only sexual partners, is a commitment many loving couples make to each other. Most people would like to be there for each other sexually, in some way. Sexual accommodation is a way to be there for your partner. Sexual accommodation can include maintenance sex. Maintenance sex can help bridge the gap of sexual differences, to meet each other's sexpectations in a limited but reasonable way, and help form a tender sexual bond between lovers.

SEXUAL ACCOMMODATION

If you are in a monogamous relationship or marriage and you have agreed to be each other's only sexual partners, and if you love your partner, you probably want to please them sexually or help them meet their sexual needs, at least some of the time. Yet let's face reality: It can be sexual drudgery to have sex when you don't feel like doing it...over and over and over again, and for hours and hours on end! No man or woman wants to feel like they have to meet her partner's *every* sexual need! With forced or implied sexual demands, a lower-desire partner can feel used and like a piece of meat.

> **Some men complain, "My wife just lies there, like a piece of dead meat!"**
> **Who do you think killed the corpse?**

No woman or man wants to feel like there is a duty to perform sexually all the time. When there's a demand to perform sexually—without a mutual agreement for sexual accommodation, without the warmth of intimacy and caring—often people's bodies stop physiologically responding to sexual demands. Sometimes men and women take creams or medications to catapult over their body's physical resistance! Men take Viagra or Cialis and women use lubricants to ready themselves physically for sex, even when they don't want it!

But there is a better solution: maintenance sex and sexual accommodation.

Most men and women would not mind, at least sometimes, to be sexually accommodating to their partners, even if they're not into sex at the moment, if it is with their full consent, for only ten minutes. Many women or men can enjoy sharing their sexual selves for 10 minutes with the partner they love in order to be sexually pleasing, if it is mutually agreed upon, not a sexual demand, AND their needs get taken care of, too. Those needs may be sexual or intimacy desires, as discussed in chapter 5, or desires for other things from their partner. For some people, they'd secretly be more than happy to share a 10 minute sexual liaison in exchange for help painting a bathroom, fixing a nice meal, or having the laundry finished and put away.

This is where some people have a problem with the Ten Minute Sexual Solution. Is sexual accommodation and negotiating for your needs to be met in your relationship or marriage okay? One therapist asked my husband and me, "How can you treat sex like it is a marital commodity, trading a lawn job for a blow job? Sex is so much more intimate and spiritual than that!" I agreed, that one's sexuality is sacred, and it can be a spiritual connection of your mind, body, and soul. Sexuality can be the most amazing and intense connection that two people can share! But is it any less sacred and special if you share it for a quickie, too? Can't you have the sacred, tantric sex on Sunday and have a 10 minute romp on Tuesday? Sharing sexual connections, even for 10 minutes, can create on ongoing bond of two souls that lasts for days! Having more frequent, although brief, sexual encounters can maintain the intimate, special sexual bond in one's relationship far better than only sharing sex once or twice a month! Sex can be like a fabulous gourmet meal, but most of us will settle for a Happy Meal on Tuesday when we're too busy and tired to cook a five course meal...and darn, those fries are pretty tasty treats!

Of course, you don't have to negotiate for any type of "commodity." You can ask for your intimacy needs to be met, such as talking, cuddling, or a backrub, without sexual demands. If that's what works for you to feel loved, receive pleasure, and want to be giving to the one you love: ASK FOR IT! Use your sexual voice, practice that sexual communication and make it work for you! The Ten Minute Sexual Solution isn't just about giving someone 10 minutes of sex, it is about asking for and receiving what you need from each other in any way, including emotionally or sexually.

You can be sexually accommodating with your partner and get little or no sexual pleasure from it, or simply enjoy the pleasure of loving them knowing that you are pleasing them. Many people can enjoy the closeness of lovemaking or plain old sex without having a sexual climax, even if it is not that sexually pleasurable. Interestingly, many lower-desire partners have said to me that they are fine with sexually accommodating their partners, but their partners are not okay with it! Specifically, some say that their partners insist that they have to have an orgasm, when they really aren't that into the sex, they don't want to, and it's okay with them not to. You need to realize that if your partner is giving you a sexual gift, you don't have to give them anything in return. It is just for you, so enjoy it! However, remember sexual accommodation is not okay if it is painful or creates discomfort.

Sexual accommodation can be acceptable if you embrace it as an activity to please your partner. You can look at it like any of a number of things you may do to please your partner, but do it without resentment. How many things does your partner do for you that take 10 minutes that they don't particularly want to do? For example, they may give you a foot rub and enjoy it for your sake, right? Also, even if you don't really get into it, you can certainly be playful, sexy, and erotic to please your partner. For example, you can give someone an erotic striptease even if you're not really in the mood for sex yourself! Or you might challenge each other: "I bet I can get you in the mood, if you'll give me five minutes of your attention!"

MASTURBATION

Talking about masturbation is a touchy subject for some couples. Many couples have never asked or talked to each other about masturbation. Yet if you have sexual differences, discussing masturbation can be important, as it can be used as a sexual option when managing sexual needs and sexpectations. Some people feel like it is none of their partner's business whether or not or how often they masturbate (or self-pleasure), as it is their private sexual business. Some people are embarrassed to tell their partners that they masturbate;

TEN MINUTE TIPS: SEXUAL ACCOMMODATION

- IF you let maintenance sex be about meeting *your* sexual needs, and not insist that your partner be sexually responsive, THEN you will be more likely to have a sexually accommodating partner. Take the demands out of sex, and enjoy yourself!

- FOR (MOSTLY) MEN: Maintenance sex doesn't mean your partner has to really, really get into it! It DOES NOT mean they have to have sexual desire or a climax! Don't make sexual demands for someone else's sexual responses or desires. If your partner doesn't get excited and scream and moan and have orgasms, let it be okay. With maintenance sex, enjoy focusing only on your own sexual sensations and pleasures for a change. Men—get over your quest for the Big O every time. Many women enjoy sexual play without having to have an orgasm! Really!

- FOR (MOSTLY) WOMEN: Get over thinking your partner has to have a "perfect erection" to have great sex! Think hands, mouth, tongues and toys. Don't get hung up on thinking that if he doesn't get an erection, that he's not attracted to you; he may just be tired and not into sex that day, not because he's not into YOU! And let it be okay that your partner doesn't climax, either! Men don't have orgasms every time, and they don't always need to have an orgasm to enjoy sex, nor have intercourse to enjoy sex, either. Really! It doesn't mean they're not attracted to you. Maybe they're just being nice to give you an orgasm before you go to bed!

they are afraid their partners will not approve. Other people know their partners masturbate, but they don't talk about it. The choice to share that information is up to you as individuals. Knowing their partner masturbates doesn't bother most people, unless there are religious prohibitions. It can also be an issue when someone is choosing to have sex with themselves or watching porn instead of having partnered sex, and someone feels deprived.

Yet discussing masturbation can help you manage your sexual differences. Imagine communicating about sex openly as you discussed sexpectations and sexual accommodation, but now talking about masturbation. Can you imagine saying to your partner, "Sorry, I don't really want to have sex today, would you mind masturbating instead?" Or, "Don't masturbate, because I want to have sex with you later today, if that's okay with you." Or maybe you're in the middle of having sex, and someone experiences sexual discomfort, so you need to stop. You might ask you partner to go ahead and masturbate instead, so they can have a sexual release. Conversely, a partner may say, "Hey, if you don't want to have sex, it's no big deal, I'll just go masturbate!" These sexual communications may seem normal, or it might seem unbelievable to you that anyone could talk like that with their partner. But why not? Remember, sex is private: It is just between you two. How you handle sex together is a very private matter, very individual, and part of being compassionate and passionate with each other.

WHAT IF ALL WE EVER HAVE IS MAINTENANCE SEX?

Frequently, I hear the complaint from one person in a couple who says, "We already have maintenance sex and that's ALL we ever have! We never have passionate lovemaking like we used to!" The Ten Minute Sexual Solution is not only about having maintenance sex: It is a program of steps that couples can use to set a foundation for a passionate, erotic, and more intimate relationship, including sex. Maintenance sex can help bridge the normal, natural differences that couples have with sexual timing and sexual differences. However, it is not the only solution to enhancing your sexual relationship. If you use all the steps of the Ten Minute Sexual Solution, and take 10 minutes a day to improve communication, have fun and play, become better friends, and embrace and accept each other, you will have a foundation for a sexual relationship that will move you beyond maintenance sex.

If sex is bland and boring and quick all the time, you are not even enjoying what I would describe as maintenance sex. Maintenance sex can be fun, exciting, pleasurable, and bonding. If you are dissatisfied with the quality of your lovemaking, go back to Sexercise #6 and discuss your sexual turn-ons and turn-offs with each other. Use what you have learned to communicate about your sexual needs and desires. Explore your relationship for hidden anger and resentments that are surfacing under your sheets. Work on being closer and more intimate outside the bedroom to improve your feelings toward each other inside the bedroom. Then, if you still are looking to spice things up in your bedroom look for a good sex book on having great sex, starting with one of the many books available on aasect.org by sex therapists.

FIVE STEPS TO MAINTENANCE SEX

1. First, complete the first three steps of *The Ten Minute Sexual Solution*, outlined in chapter 3. Work on sexual communication and talk to each other about what you want, including what you want outside of the bedroom. Take a look at your relationship beyond the bedroom, and assess the intimacy in your marriage. It may be that your relationship needs to improve in one or more areas of intimacy to feel closer and stir up sexual passion. Next, take a look at the anger or resentments in your marriage: Is there a wedge between you that needs to be removed? Start with the One Month Program of *The Ten Minute Sexual Solution* (chapter 3), taking 10 minutes a day to work on your relationship for one month, before you practice maintenance sex.

2. Second, directly discuss the differences in your sexual desire, including your sexual cycles (Sexercise #11) and sexpectations.

3. Third, discuss using maintenance sex to bridge the gap of differences between you. If one of you wants to have sex every day and the other wants sex once a week or less, discuss how often you might use maintenance sex to increase your sexual frequency. For example, you

> may agree to continue making love on Saturday night and agree to
> have maintenance sex on one weekday night once a week.
>
> 4. Share your sexual expectations for maintenance sex. For example, for
>   some couples, maintenance sex might mean giving oral sex to their
>   partner or using manual stimulation to simply "get someone off." For
>   another couple, it might mean having sexual intercourse, with the
>   understanding that it lasts 10 minutes, not for an hour. Use Sexercise
>   #6 (your sexual turn-ons and turn-offs) for suggestions.
>
> 5. When initiating maintenance sex, develop a system for communicat-
>   ing how important it is for you to have sex. Use the rating system
>   described in Sexercise #4, Developing Your Sexual Voice, to tell each
>   other where you are at sexually. When you are way out of sexual sync
>   or someone is desperate, use maintenance sex to bridge the gap.

How Does Maintenance Sex Work with the Ten Minute Sexual Solution?

The Ten Minute Sexual Solution is taking 10 minutes to spend time
alone for physically loving one another, once you have taken the steps
to create a foundation of sexual communication and intimacy for
maintenance sex. You can start immediately to increase the sexual frequency in your marriage by including maintenance sex in your sexual repertoire. For some couples, after the first two or three years of their
sexual relationship, about 50 percent of their sexual activity is maintenance sex, while the other 50 percent is longer lasting, passionate lovemaking. Some couples wait to have sex until they have time for longer
lasting lovemaking and fireworks sex. Including maintenance sex into
your sexual activity can double your sex life immediately!

Sexual marathons are fabulous, but every sexual experience can't
be a peak sexual experience. One of the best things about sex isn't
just the ultimate physical experience; it's about being wanted and
loved. Everyone wants to be wanted, even for a few minutes.

> **Maintenance sex is about being loving and caring to your
> partner...for just 10 minutes.**

(Almost) Famous Ten Minute Maintenance Sex Solutions

Maintenance sex is not simply having a meaningless quickie. Here are some awesome ideas for great 10 minute sexual interludes that are fun and fulfilling.

- Sex in the shower (the water will get cold anyway)
- Sex in the fileroom at work (it really does happen!)
- Sex in an airplane
- Making out in your minivan
- Sex at your parents' house
- Sex during the commercials
- Sex during halftime
- Sex while the kids play next door at the neighbors
- Sex with the vibrator, being held by your partner
- Sex on your lunch hour
- Sex in the morning before work
- Sex while live-in mom/dad is having a nap
- Sex at 3 A.M.
- Sex while the baby is napping
- Blow jobs (almost) anywhere
- Oops! Sex that didn't last that long, but it is was OK for one of you

8

Creating Sexual Desire

Amazingly, every week women and men come into my office with the same complaint: They don't want sex! Low sexual desire is the most common sexual problem and the major cause of sexless relationships. Whether you are the one with low sexual desire or the partner who desperately wants your partner to want you—creating sexual desire and learning to love sex are essential to changing your sex life. Understanding and changing low sexual desire for some people **can happen** by taking a different approach to creating sexual desire—a new approach to low sexual desire introduced in this chapter!

New approaches to creating sexual desire are a part of the Ten Minute Sexual Solution to change sexual desire in a lower-desire partner, and to help couples shrink the gap of sexual differences. Part I of this chapter will focus on creating sexual desire using the new approach to understanding and changing sexual desire. Part II of this chapter focuses on creating sexual by understanding different types of low sexual desire and learning to enjoy sexual pleasure, with easy, step-by-step, straight-forward solutions for some individuals.

PART I: A NEW APPROACH TO CREATING SEXUAL DESIRE

Most women and men with low sexual desire **want to want sex**—
to feel sexual, sensual, and desire sex "like other people do." Having
even one peak sexual experience that makes them smile, sweetly, in
the middle of the day, for no other reason than to have a deep sigh-
ing moment remembering sexual passion is an elusive goal for many
people. Instead, people are thinking and feeling:

- "What is wrong with me?"
- "Why don't I even care about sex?"
- "Why doesn't s/he want sex?"
- "It doesn't make sense, almost every time we have sex we both love it!"
- "Why can't I seem to want sex or enjoy sex, like the mag- azines describe, like my sister/brother/friends and even *mother* describes?"
- "Why don't I feel how my partner wants me to feel?"
- "I could live the rest of my life without sex."
- "I want that look in my eyes, that step in my walk, where someone looks at me and whispers, 'Wow, s/he must have gotten laid last night!'"

THE FACTS ABOUT SEXUAL DESIRE[1,2]

- One third of women report lacking sexual desire.
- Up to 15 percent of men have low sexual desire.
- 20 percent of couples have a sexless marriage (10 times a year or less, or never).
- 15 percent of couples have sex twice a month or less.
- 50 percent of marriages have a problem with low sexual desire at some point.

A NEW PERSPECTIVE ON SEXUAL DESIRE

A new perspective, particularly about women and sexual desire, can
change a couple's entire sexual relationship! This section focuses

primarily on women, as currently, more information is known at this point about women and low sexual desire than men. Understanding about sexual desire has derived from research on "The Sexual Response Cycle." Theories and research on how sex works have taught people (including sex therapists) that the sexual response cycle, or how people respond to sex, goes like this: First people have sexual desire, then sexual excitement and/or arousal, then orgasms[3]. This model has become a cultural understanding of "how sex works" for the last four decades. Research has trickled down over the years to modern media and magazines, where "tips to feel sexy" have become the golden ticket to great sex and relationships. Women wait, and wait, and wait until the first feeling of sexual desire happens to them, to feel "sexy" and want to have sex. Men wait until they feel sexual stirrings, or have partial erections, before they'll consider initiating sex. After all, that's the formula for sex, right? You feel sexy, you feel sensuous, you wait until you're "in the mood," and then you are ready for sex, right? Yet, many busy women (and some men) **NEVER** (or seldom) think about sex. They don't get "horny." So, they rarely initiate sex, and they avoid any physical or sexual contact that would lead to sex.

Let me introduce you to a new way of thinking about how many people experience sexual feelings. Some individuals need to experience physical touch, including cuddling, caressing, kissing, and sexual touch **FIRST,** and **THEN** they experience sexual excitement, with sexual desire **FOLLOWING** the feelings of sexual arousal. In other words, some people have to get turned on first, before they feel like being turned on.

> **Some women need to experience sexual feelings**
> *first,* **and** *then* **they feel sexual desire.**

> **Sometimes people don't experience a feeling until they're feeling the experience.**

Some people need to experience an intimate, sexual moment first, before they feel the sexual moment and then desire sex. When women and men wait for women to "be in the mood," or feel sexual desire, or want to have sex, they often wait a very long time. Changing expectations, sexpections, and changing the way men and women approach sex, can completely change a couple's sexual relationship.

OLD FORMULA FOR SEX:
Sexual desire, then sexual arousal, then orgasm

NEW FORMULA FOR SEX:
Sexual arousal, then sexual desire, then orgasm

As one of my clients said, "It doesn't make sense, almost every time we make love we both love it! So, why doesn't she want to have sex more often?" The problem is that the lower-desire partner doesn't think about sex very often. However, for some people, after touch starts, perhaps in a nonsexual way, with kissing, touching, ravishing, and rubbing against each other, THEN they feel sexual desire.

> **After physical touching begins, many otherwise low sexual desire individuals do NOT WANT YOU TO STOP!**

When the lower-desire partner begins to physically respond to touching, they often do feel sexual desire and they want to keep going until they have more intense sexual touching, including touch that leads to sexual arousal and orgasm. For many "lower-desire" people, it is not that they don't desire sex, it's just that they don't feel sexual desire or think about sex until after they feel physical touch and get excited. In other words, they need to have sexual arousal first. In addition, some women experience "arousal," even without physical touching, when they have deep emotional intimacy with their partners, such as after a particularly touching talk about a personal subject. Some women who have not experienced sexual desire in a long time begin to have feelings of desire following deep intimate sharing (see Sexercise #10 for an example), as well as direct physical touch and stimulation.

THE SEXUAL TOUCHING PARADOX

The old formula of how sex works—waiting for sexual desire to happen, and then approaching physical and sexual touch—has a negative, paradoxical effect on a relationship that, in fact, decreases sexual desire. Many people who don't feel sexual desire also avoid sexual touch. In fact, they avoid ANY touch! Anyone in a relationship with low sexual frequency knows that this is true: any physical contact, including kissing, hugging, touching, cuddling when you go to bed, or even touching each other when you pass in the hallway, is avoided. Paradoxically, the less physical contact you have, the less likely you are going to feel any sexual feelings, and the less likely you are going to EVER experience sexual desire!

> **The more you avoid touch to avoid sex, the less likely you are to experience sexual desire!**

PHYSICAL TOUCH AND SEXUAL DESIRE:

JESSI AND JORDAN'S STORY

Jessi was Hispanic and she came from a very "touchy-feely" family. If you went to see her family, you got a lot of hugs. In the beginning of her marriage to Jordan, they used to touch each other all the time, sit on each other's lap, and sometimes, as she said it, "Gross out our friends with the way we had our hands all over each other." Jordan came from a family where he was the only child. His mom and dad were more reserved, and they didn't hug or kiss each other much, except at weddings and funerals. While Jordan did like to touch and kiss, it certainly was not as much as his wife of nine years.

Jessi liked touching more than Jordan. She also liked cuddling and even holding hands more than he did. Over the course of their marriage, they had had two kids. Both are in elementary school now. In the past two years, Jessi said that Jordan just stopped liking being touched all the time. If she hugged him, he'd cringe. If she tried to kiss him, he didn't open his mouth and it was a peck. If she tried to pull him over in the bed next to her, he'd turn away and go to sleep. Jessi thought that maybe it was Jordan's family background, but that didn't make sense because he used to love touching her! Jessi felt very rejected. She felt unattractive. She wondered if her husband loved her anymore.

Jordan told Jessi he loved her very much. In therapy, he said that he and his wife got along very well and were the best of friends, they just didn't have sex or touch very often. Jessi said she felt like they were very good roommates and parents together but she wished they could have more sex, too. Over the past two years of their marriage, their sex life had dwindled down to having sex once a month or less. Going for several weeks without having sex had happened more than a few times. Jessi just didn't understand it! She was an attractive, sexy woman, with a pretty hot body. Jessi said every time they made love, they both enjoyed it immensely! They both gave and received pleasure and felt so good during lovemaking and afterwards! Jessi simply didn't understand why Jordan didn't want more sex. She wondered if he was gay, or maybe having an affair. Embarrassingly, she had hired a private investigator, who found nothing and cost Jessi $3,000 to report that Jordan went to a book store a couple of times, alone, and bought a business book and two children's books for their girls.

Jordan reported that he simply didn't think about sex anymore. He was a teacher, but he spent most of his free time picking up the kids from school, or grading papers and getting ready for class the next day. Jessi was in banking and worked long hours, hoping not to get laid off, like a lot of her colleagues who had been downsized. On top of work, Jordan helped the girls with homework, as well as cooked dinner, although Jessi did help with dinner and dishes most nights. Jordan was a bit of a perfectionist, though, and always wanted to get the dishes and laundry and house picked up before he could go to bed at night. Interestingly, Jessi said Jordan was like "the woman" because he did so much around the house. That was why she thought he might be gay. Jordan was a great husband, but he just didn't have any interest in or energy for sex. By the end of a day, Jordan simply felt exhausted and never felt sexual desire. In the past few years, he started going to bed right after the girls went to bed. Jordan did say that he did enjoy making love with Jessi, and she was a sexy, wonderful lover, but just the thought of having sex seemed like too much work and energy.

Jordan was one of those people, who did, in fact, like sex and even LOVE making love with his wife, once sex got started. The problem was it rarely got started because he never felt any sexual desire. And he avoided sex and any physical touch, and went to bed early every night. On the weekends, he was up, out of bed early, getting the girls to practice, or working on the yard.

Jordan was a great guy, a good husband, who never had a role model for how to be a "lover." His parents were never close, and he thought they might have had sex twice in their life: conceiving him and his sister. Jordan was definitely not gay, and he was very attracted to his wife. Jordan was a bit obsessive about work, sometimes spending more time on his classwork than with his wife, as well as housework, making sure everything got finished every night. He just didn't think about sex because he was too task-oriented. Interestingly, people who are over-thinkers and obsessive, appear more likely to experience sexual desire *after* arousal, because they don't stop to think about sex.

Jordan and Jessi were introduced to a new way to approach sexual desire, realizing that some people just don't feel it or have it until after physical touch or until after sex starts. They agreed to try Sexercise #9: A Touching Exercise, to start. Jordan agreed to allow physical touch between them again. Jessi agreed that if Jordan didn't want sex, it was okay. Even though Jessi had gotten upset in the past, if she got excited from hugging or kissing and it didn't lead to sex, she agreed to stop putting sexual demands on every kind of physical touch. Jordan had to learn to trust Jessi, so he could feel safe starting touch and stopping if he wanted to or if he was too tired. This trust allowed him to feel safe and relaxed, enjoying touch enough that he could experience sexual desire.

After a few times of practicing nonsexual touching, Jordan began to feel some sexual desire! In fact, the third time they completed the sexercise, they made love—when *Jordan* insisted, despite the "rules." A little while after their success, Jordan agreed to try maintenance sex, too. For Jordan, he was too tired to consider having 30 minutes or an hour of lovemaking very often. Yet, he was open to taking 10 minutes for touching, really just thinking he was doing it for Jessi, to have maintenance sex. Jordan was surprised that almost all of the time, he got turned on from the touching at the beginning of a session of maintenance sex, and had feelings of sexual desire return, too! In fact, Jessi reported that they both had sexual pleasure every time they tried just 10 minutes of sex, even though Jessi didn't have an orgasm every time. Jordan agreed to try to have maintenance sex once a week, even if he wasn't in the mood, to see if he would respond to physical touching, and to make Jessi happier by being her sexual partner. Jordan really needed to take time out, to make time, for a sexual relationship in his marriage, which was new and strange to him. After a few months, Jessi was very happy with their renewed, more consistent sexual relationship, although she consistently had to remind him to come to bed and spend time with her. For Jessi, it was an important change to realize she was wanted by her husband, even if she had to remind him to spend time with her.

THE NEW APPROACH TO SEXUAL DESIRE AND THE TEN MINUTE SEXUAL SOLUTION

So how does this new approach to sexual desire fit in with the Ten Minute Sexual Solution? First, couples have to remember the first few steps of *The Ten Minute Sexual Solution*. You have to have the foundation of communication and intimacy to set the stage for creating sexual desire and sharing maintenance sex. Jessi and Jordan had a very close friendship and good communication already, they just didn't touch or have sex. The key was to start touching again, and to introduce maintenance sex later.

Couples who have stopped touching or avoid touch can give each other permission to begin to have physical and intimate interaction again. Make sure you agree, as a couple, that it really is okay to physically touch and even be sexually playful, without having it be a demand for sex. When lower-desire partners feel they can touch you, without worrying that it has to lead to sex, they will want to touch more! The more touching you share, the more likely, in the long-run, that it will lead to sexual desire and sexual feelings. So start being more physically playful with each other! Let it be okay to for someone to play with you with touch and then turn around and say, "No, I don't want sex, I just wanted to feel your body!" Remember, at all times: Use your sexual voice! Every moment of touch, and even sexual touch, does not have to lead to sex, just as it was for most couples in the beginning of their relationship. Many couples remember having "spontaneous sex," in the beginning of their sexual relationship, when in fact, the sex followed lots of nonsexual touching. Sex didn't come spontaneously: Physical touch created sexual desire!

CREATING SEXUAL TRANSITIONS

For busy couples, understanding how people feel sexual desire, then creating sexual moments first, can change your sex life. Women often need a transition from life to wife to sex life before they even think about sex, and in order to experience sexual desire. Creating new sexual scripts can start by creating sexual transitions. For some couples, discovering a different way to approach sex, using sexual transitions and creating a sexual moment with physical interaction and touching, is enough to lead to sex.

> **Most women (and some men) need to make a transition from their *life*... to their sex life.**

Getting from life to your sex life is a challenge for many couples. Some couples create personal rituals to make transitions from their life to their sex life. Some couples simply use their own personal sexual signature to initiate sex. Some individuals try to find the window of sexual opportunity and pray and hope and wish to find a way through the hoops to sex. Creating your own sexual transitions as a couple, will help you move from partners to lovers more easily and often.

TEN MINUTE TIPS TO TRANSITION TO YOUR SEX LIFE

- Take a hot bubble bath together.
- Turn off the lights and light candles in the bedroom.
- Turn on soft/romantic/or sexy music.
- Offer to give or receive a hot oil backrub—no strings attached.
- Go to bed together, even if it's early, and cuddle.
- Put on lingerie/ask your partner to change to sexy clothing.
- Ask your partner to makeout.
- Turn off the computer and put away work.
- Open a bottle of wine or make some tea and sit down to talk.
- Give/receive a foot rub.
- Passionately kiss your partner.
- Put the kids in bed early (turn the clocks back 30 minutes to fool them into an early bedtime, if you're desperate and tired).
- Offer oral sex, no strings attached.

SEXERCISE #12

CREATING SEXUAL TRANSITIONS

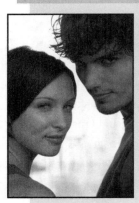

Using the ten minute tips for creating sexual transitions, take 10 minutes to create a one of your own. Build your own sexual signature as a couple to create a transition from life to your sex life, together. Try at least two different things over the next two weeks. At first, you might feel awkward and silly, but after you practice transitions together, they will come more naturally to you as a couple. Practice the art of being seductive, as well, allowing transitions to be erotic encounters!

PART II: CREATING SEXUAL DESIRE

YOUR SEXUAL SELF: PRIMARY LOW SEXUAL DESIRE

Have you EVER enjoyed sex? This section is for people who have never experienced what they would call sexual desire or sexual pleasure. There are two types of sexual desire problems: primary problems and secondary problems. A primary problem is when you have never felt any sexual desire or don't think you have, ever. Yet the vast majority of people that I see fall into the second category: They once felt sexual desire, but they don't any more. The vast majority of people have, at some point, felt sexual desire and experienced sexual excitement, whether it was alone or with someone else. Then gradually, but sometimes suddenly, they stop feeling any sexual desire at all. Some people report they have never had any sexual desire, but closer examination reveals that they often don't know how to define sexual feelings, as with the next case.

"JENA"

Jena was a beautiful young woman in her early thirties. She had been married for about six years to an extremely dull man called "Howard." Jena came in for therapy because she felt no sexual desire, and in fact, she never had orgasms or sexual pleasure with her husband. Jena and Howard both worked full time in the same type of medical field and had met in college.

While it sounds mean to say that Howard was dull, it is relevant, as it carried over to his marriage. Howard went to work, went home, read history books, and wouldn't allow a TV in his house, as he thought it would "dull the mind" (how ironic!), and his only hobby was bird hunting in the spring. Sexually, Howard was a missionary type of guy: You're on a mission to have sex because you're supposed to and need to, it is in the missionary position, but you know it's going to be a short mission. Howard was a fast shooter, so to speak, having a problem with premature ejaculation.

Jena didn't have a dysfunctional sexual past. She was a "good girl" raised in a good Southern Baptist Church, and had married a "good guy." Jena was, technically, a virgin when they got married. She had dated and messed around a bit, but never went all the way until her wedding night.

Jena came in for sex therapy because she didn't have any sexual desire for her husband. She didn't get anything out of sex, and she felt that sex, as brief as it was, was sexual drudgery. She also reported that she didn't have orgasms. Jena had never "touched herself down there." She was brought up to believe that masturbation was a sin, so she "never did that and was never going to, so don't tell me to do that!"

It was a concern that Jena was unwilling to explore her own sexual feelings by herself. Then, we spoke a little more. It turns out that Jena actually DID have sexual feelings and sexual responses...but it wasn't with Howard. But they didn't count, she said.

Actually, at least a couple of times a week, maybe more, since Jena was a little girl, she would use the sheets on her bed, to rub them between her legs, back and forth, and have an orgasm. Even to this day, she would enjoy the feeling and look forward to the pleasure of rubbing herself with the her bed pillow, sometimes vigorously, between her legs, after Howard went to work early in the morning and before she quite awoke, a few times a week. She never told Howard about this, and she wasn't "masturbating" (since she didn't touch herself). Because she didn't get any pleasure from sex or count those orgasms, she came in to see me, worried that she had no sexual desire.

Jena, obviously, did in fact have sexual desire and she was wired physically for sex, which was fabulous as far as I was concerned. Jena thought that there was something terribly wrong with her sexually, when in fact, she was quite functional sexually, but not in the way that she **defined** "sex" or sexual desire, and not in the way that she wanted to be.

Jena's therapy was largely a huge success! After she revealed that she did, in fact, have sexual feelings, and that she did, in fact, have a capacity to enjoy sexual pleasure, she simply needed to learn to own that and then share her sexual self with her husband. The very good news was that Jena did, indeed, have a sexual self: She was a sexual person, but she did not have a sexual identity. Jena did not know how to talk about sex or be sexual with Howard. In fact, she was embarrassed about sex.

Sex therapy helped Jena become quite successful in developing a sexual voice. She learned how to talk about sex openly in therapy and learned to feel comfortable with the idea of being a sexual person. Jena later opened up to her husband, told him what she liked sexually, and asked him to share with her sexually, for the first time. Fortunately, Howard listened and let Jena guide him, sexually, and then later, socially, as well. Howard also got treated for premature ejaculation, and he began to enjoy sex more. It really just took some understanding about what was "sexual" to accept her sexual self, and ultimately explore who she was and express what she wanted, sexually speaking. Jena, like many women and some men, needed to first feel comfortable with her own sexual identity. After their huge success, Howard also began to listen to her about social and entertainment matters, as well: They got a TV, they had a child, and they joined a local golf course/country club!

For some reason, Jena did not define her self-pleasuring on a regular basis as part of her sexual identity. She only defined her sexual self as who she was with someone else: her husband. On her own, Jena was very much enjoying sex! Often, clients don't define or don't want to define their sexual responses as being "sexual." I know this sounds really weird, but it's true. I have had many clients diagnosed with primary sexual desire problems who did, indeed, have sexual experiences in their past, whether they were wanted or unwanted, by themselves or with partners (including same-sex partners at young ages) during which they felt sexual responses and even sexual pleasure. For some reason those feelings were repulsive or not "named" as sexual response. For Jena, she couldn't admit to her sexual feelings because it would be defined as masturbation, which was sinful to her, but they were there!

If you've got a "primary sexual desire" problem, explore your present and your past to see if there is or was a time you feel or felt sexual response. If you have, work to own and accept these feelings, and you can build on them—on your own first, then later with your partner, if and when you would like. If you have never had any sexual feelings or you would like to explore some inklings of feelings you currently have, we'll discuss in detail in chapter 9 how to mentally and physically explore (or find!) your sexual feelings. If you would like to have sexual desire, it is very important for you to explore your sexual feelings and responses for yourself, to create your sexual identity and want to be a sexual person.

If you once had sexual feelings or responses but you don't now, you may have turned off your sexual switch, and/or have "secondary sexual problems."

YOUR SEXUAL SELF: SECONDARY LOW SEXUAL DESIRE

As stated earlier, most people with sexual desire problems once had sexual desire, but somewhere along the way, it was lost. Finally, here is your guide on how to find it! Remember, at this point, we are still focusing solely on you. Focus on your sexual self, not on how you feel when you are with someone else, but on your own thoughts and feelings about sex. With secondary sexual desire problems, the goal is to find out what caused you to stop thinking about or wanting sex. Or, in other words, you want to know what made you turn off your sexual switch, as a child or as an adult.

Did You TURN OFF Your Sexual Switch?

REASONS WHY PEOPLE HAVE TURNED OFF THEIR SEXUAL SWITCH AT AN EARLY AGE

- Sexual traumas, such as sexual abuse and incest
- Strict religious past regarding the sins of sexual thought, action, or masturbation
- Parental instruction against masturbation/ getting "caught"
- Unusual exposure to sex, such as viewing the "primal scene" (seeing your parents having sex) or pornography

If you have had a problem with sexual abuse in your past, and you believe it might be affecting your sexuality now, I recommend reading Wendy Maltz's book, *The Sexual Healing Journey*, or Mike Lew's book, *Victims No Longer: The Classic Guide for Men Recovering from Sexual Child Abuse (Second Edition).*

Often, adults are not aware of when or how their sexual switch was turned off as a child. Adults who were sexually abused as children often have sexual desire problems, but certainly not all. In fact, only one half of adult survivors of sexual abuse report that they have long-lasting sexual effects from sexual abuse. On the other hand, sexual abuse can be a debilitating trauma that strongly impacts sexuality. If you feel trauma has affected your life, or you've had trauma but don't know if it is related to your sexual problem, seek a professional consultation with a sex therapist. With some sexual abuse survivors it takes intensive psychotherapy and/or hypnotherapy to pinpoint an event or time that caused a shutting down of one's sexual self. Still, it is very possible to turn the switch back on and reclaim your sexuality.

REASONS WHY PEOPLE HAVE TURNED OFF THEIR SEXUAL SWITCH AS AN ADULT

- Sexual difficulties or sexual dysfunctions that make people avoid sex: premature ejaculation, inability to have orgasms, erection problems, vaginismus, pain with intercourse, delayed ejaculation
- Sexual assault as an adult
- Relationship problems
- Stress-/work-related problems
- Postpartum depression and depression in general
- Alcoholism and other addictions and diseases, such as diabetes
- Medications, such as antidepressants

Sexual problems kill sexual desire. Basically, something happens sexually that ranges from uncomfortable to very anxiety–provoking. Often, if you have a sexual problem, you try and try and try to solve it. Every time it recurs, there's a huge moment of emotional and sexual anxiety, and it makes you want to avoid sex. The good news is that if you have a secondary sexual problem, and you turned off your sexual switch, it is likely that you can turn it back on, if you can identify what happened. Many times, people know exactly why they lost sexual desire, and the most common reasons are relationship problems. The Ten Minute Sexual Solution can help couples reclaim or create sexual desire by improving their relationship through communication and intimacy.

YOUR SEXUAL SELF: SITUATIONAL SEXUAL DESIRE PROBLEMS

Situational low sexual desire is when in some situations you feel desire, while in others, you don't. As stated above, one example is when men or women feel sexual desire and choose to masturbate regularly, but have no desire for sex with their partner. Another example of low sexual desire is when a person has no desire for sex with their partner, but seeks extramarital affairs and feels a great deal of sexual desire. If you have situational sexual desire, then you don't have a problem with low sexual desire from a medical perspective. You have low sexual desire due to relationship problems or for individual psycho-social-sexual reasons.

Situational low sexual desire can sometimes be easily explained, while in other cases it is highly complex. An easily understood situation is when the lower-desire partner is in an emotionally abusive relationship. In such a relationship, the lower-desire partner may be constantly criticized, judged, controlled, and even demeaned. In response, he or she feels resentment, anger, and even indifference to a point of not loving or even liking his or her partner any longer. In sex therapy, the lower-desire partner may come in for help for having no sexual desire. In cases of intense anger, resentment, and/or a lack of attraction, it is easily understood that one feels no sexual desire. Often, they will feel like there is something wrong because they never think about sex or want it. In fact, it may be very puzzling when they have felt sexual desire in their past, but it diminished or they now feel sexually dead. Quite the contrary, it is normal to have no sexual desire toward someone who is abusive! In this case, the low sexual desire is specific to this situation or partner.

Complex situational low sexual desire can benefit from a consultation from a therapist. Sometimes an outside observer can quickly pinpoint the situational sexual desire problem that seems so perplexing to you. On the other hand, reasons can be a result of complex psycho-sexual factors. One example of this is the person who can only feel high sexual desire or intense sexual response in a situation where there is low emotional commitment. Or when there is high emotional commitment, there is mysteriously low sexual desire. In these cases, complex psycho-sexual factors are at play, and a sex therapist is recommended.

Sexual Intimacy with Yourself

Whether your sexual desire problem is primary, secondary, or situational, it is important to work on creating a new sexual identity for yourself, in order to create sexual desire. A major part of this process is to begin with intimacy with yourself, in order to explore your sexual thoughts, feelings, and the sexual behaviors that interest and excite you and turn you on. Most people think of intimacy as being with only another person. While that may be true, you need to start by being intimate with yourself first, to discover and define what you like and what is close to your heart before you can share that with another person.

Your sexual identity provides the building blocks for the creation of sexual desire. This chapter gave you the basics of understanding sexual desire. The next chapters provide essential information to teach you how to create sexual desire for yourself, including how to have different types of sexual pleasure. Imagine creating a sexual identity that includes loving sex, erotic fantasies, orgasms, and sharing your sexual self with your partner, too.

9

Ten Minutes a Day: For Women

Where are you, sexually speaking? Do you like sex? Are you comfortable with sex? Do you feel pretty good about your sexuality, but you just need a tune-up? Do you think things are going fine with you sexually, but your relationship has some roadblocks due to resentments, anger, fatigue, time, privacy, or communicating about sex? Do you feel like you are missing something sexually, but you can't put it into words? Maybe you would you like to figure out how to enjoy sex more? Do you feel sexually pressured by your partner? Or do you have a problem with your partner seeming to always demand sex, and you simply don't know what to do?

If so, would you like to love sex, for yourself? Much of this chapter is written for the lower-desire woman, which is the majority of women, although some lower-desire men may relate to it. Women with higher desire may relate more with the next chapter, for higher-desire men, but the end of this chapter highlights information for higher-desire women, as well.

This chapter is to help women unleash, reclaim, or begin to discover your sexual power as a woman. Why not unleash your personal sexual power? Not for anyone else, but for you! To have the Ten Minute Sexual Solution work for you as a woman, learn to reclaim or discover your own sexuality identity. This chapter will teach you to enjoy sex: to feel sensuous, sexy, to "feel like a woman," to enjoy more pleasure and develop your own sexual identity. If you let go and reclaim, or discover your full sexual power, you might find that you actually enjoy, look forward to, and want sex. If you had a mind-blowing orgasm every time you had sex, *as most men do*, would you want it more? Do you remember from chapter 1 that only 29 percent of women, but 75 percent of men ALWAYS have orgasms during sex[1]? If you had more reliable orgasms, you might look forward to sex more, too! If sex wasn't just meeting a physical need, no more exciting than eating unsalted crackers when you were hungry, but instead, a powerful, erotic connection between you and your partner, would you want it more? If you could get a satisfying sexual release and reliably have pleasurable orgasms in 10 minutes, would you enjoy using the Ten Minute Sexual Solution?

Up to half of women have a problem with low sexual desire or sexual arousal during their lives, and half of couples have problems with different sexual desires. This chapter is aimed at helping women who experience sexual desire problems or would like to learn how to have multiple orgasms or experience female ejaculation. Women, if your sexual partner has a stronger sex drive than you, before judging them too harshly and giving up on sexual compatibility, why not first really try to embrace sex for yourself and get more pleasure from your own sexuality? Embrace your true sexual self and share your unique erotic nature with your partner! You may come to understand that your man's sex drive is often a biological need, not a power or control trip. As sexist a statement as it may be, it's simply true that men in their teens, twenties, and thirties often DO have a strong sexual drive that outpaces women of that same age group. Part of this is male testosterone and biological sex drive, but a good part of this difference in sex drives is due to women not claiming their full sexual potential until they are in their thirties and forties.

Women have been taught to be nonsexual and have learned many incorrect facts about their own sexuality. Part of the problem is cultural messages that women receive about sex that suppress their natural sexual drives and individual sexual exploration. Women may experience their "sexual peak" 20 years after men because it takes them 20 years to unlearn destructive beliefs about sex. For example, if you are 18 years old—the age men have their "sexual peak"—and you are a young woman who loves sex, you'll probably be considered a "slut" or a "whore." Most women shut down their sexuality to meet cultural, religious, or family expectations. At 18 years old you are still supposed to be a chaste virgin, never even thinking of sex until you are married, right? Even young women who *are* sexually active report less sexual pleasure from sex than men! God knows, if you're "immoral" enough to be having sex, you better not be enjoying it! How many 18-year-old young men aren't enjoying sex and having orgasms because they're feeling immoral and sinful?

THE FIRST KEY TO CREATING YOUR SEXUAL IDENTITY

First, I'm going to share with you a very important sexual secret: The key to creating sexual desire is to stop having sex for someone else, to stop being nonsexual because of someone else, and to begin to create you own sexual voice, your own sexual identity, your own sexual relationship, and—regardless of the circumstances of your life—to awaken and embrace your true sexual self.

Put aside the sexual demands, negative comments, or feelings about how you *never* want sex or *never* have sex or *never* look sexy or *never whatever!* For now, just focus on sex for yourself. If it is difficult for you to focus on your sexual self, or even clear your mind to think about sex, don't worry! This is a guide to help you get your sexual self tuned in and turned on!

As a sex therapist, I am not in the business of making people have sex who don't want to. I am here to help you discover, uncover, develop, and create your own sexual identity, for yourself FIRST…and then you can decide to share it with someone, if and when you desire. I wrote this chapter for YOU—the one with the lower sexual desire, the one who may be feeling pressured to have sex for someone else, the one who may want to be sexual and feel sexual, but just doesn't, and may not even know why! Or if you DO know why, you don't know how to change it, or IF you want to change it. I know and you know that your sexual being can thrive or die in any particular relationship, so we will work on helping you thrive sexually within your relationship, too. But first, any sexual intimacy starts with intimacy with yourself.

THREE STEPS TO SEXUAL INTIMACY WITH YOURSELF

1. Clear your mind.
2. Mind your body.
3. Practice self-pleasuring to connect your mind and body.

THE SEXLESS MIND

- "I don't WANT to think about sex…it just makes me feel sad and I don't enjoy it anyway."
- "I don't think about sex much, but when we do it, I really enjoy it."
- "I don't think about sex much, but it's ok, even though I don't have orgasms."

Do you ever think about sex? If not, is it because the sex is lousy, or because you're too busy thinking or obsessing about other things to bother? When you do have sex, do you enjoy it? Do you feel sexual pleasure, do you have orgasms, or really get something out of it so that you'll look forward to it? Or does a problem with sex make you NOT want sex? Do you shut off your sexual desire?

TURNING ON YOUR MIND

You have to clear your mind to clear the way to find your sexual self. It takes some work. Your sexual self is sometimes so deep inside you, or gets buried deep inside you, it's like an antique that's been sitting on a shelf for so long that it has to be dusted off and polished to find out that it's a treasure.

Often a lack of sexual desire is simply due to having too many things to think about, beside sex. This is very common for women, and happens to some men, too. For most men, it is very hard to believe that women often go an entire day without thinking about sex…AND they might even go a week, or a month, without really having serious sexual thoughts or sexual fantasies! One barrier to sexual thoughts and feelings is memories of anxiety-ridden episodes of unsuccessful sexual interludes with your partner (or from your past). However, a very large barrier to sexual desire is the obsessive overthinking of life's tasks, details, and work.

> **A major barrier to sexual desire for women, and some men, is a distracted or obsessive mind that thinks about everything else first and sex last, if ever.**

While I find that almost everyone can benefit from learning to clear their mind and make a transition from everyday life to sexual thoughts, some people tend to be even more obsessive or distracted and NOT think about sex. People who fall into this category tend to be people who worry a lot, are workaholics, hyper, perfectionist, people with ADD and ADHD, and people who are diagnosed with or seen as "obsessive-compulsive" or "anal." A common scenario is a woman doing laundry and cleaning the kitchen at 10 P.M., while making cookies for her child's school the next day. This woman is not thinking about sex that night! Some people are especially obsessive and distracted, and sexual thoughts don't enter their mind. If this is you—you are going to have to take extra time with this section. If this doesn't help—you might need professional help to tune in and get turned on, whether with a psychotherapist or a psychiatrist.

Most women and some men need to learn to stop the world and pay attention to themselves and their body, for a change. Such men and women are often sensitive people who are doers and givers and put other people first. For the first time in your life, or for the first time in a long time, put yourself first.

THE SEXUAL POSITION TRANSITION

You need a transition from your position as second: second to your boss, second to your parents, second to your children, second to your housework, and even second to your car! You, my dearest reader, need to become first! But in order to become first, you have to make a transition to first place. You have to do what you must to become your sexual self…to start by making a transition from the person who serves another person, place, or thing, to one who serves her sexual self.

"THE LIST"

Often people think of priorities in life as a hierarchy. People like to think of their priorities, proudly, in an order of importance, such as: God, family, work, school, friends, and hobbies. The truth is that even though we may value all of those elements of The List in some moral, righteous way, life simply does not allow us to put all of our values first at all times! The truth is that if a 3-year-old has an earache in the middle of the night and is screaming with pain, the number one priority for every person who is now awake in that house is to get immediate medical care—even if work or church are supposed to come in the morning.

Women tend to put themselves at the end of this theoretical priority list. Busy with life, work, church, school, and children, a woman's individual sexual feelings are often at the bottom of a list of other things to do first. Sometimes there are no choices but to attend to other things, such as an earache. But sometimes women need to make a transition to putting themselves, including their sexuality, first, without guilt.

Guilt kills genuine sexual desire.

Abandon your belief in judging yourself because you put yourself first at some times, even above all other things on your imaginary hierarchy of life's values. Stop thinking about what you have to or should do or must do, especially during sex. I can't tell you how many women have told me that when they are lying in bed, receiving oral sex, looking at the ceiling, they are thinking that they need to clean the kitchen floor, or get a report written, or hurry up to get up and fix brownies. Give yourself a break! Make a sexual position transition and think about sex!

MAKING YOUR BREAK

If you want to get to where you want to go from where you are, then you need to learn how to make a break. After all, we are talking about finding your sexual self, right?

You will need a mental health tool box. If you haven't got one yet, don't worry...I'm going to teach you how to create one, right now! Every one has stress, everyone has worries, everyone is distracted by the details of life, and forgets to live, to breathe—and to breathe life into their sex life! Your mental health tool box MUST include ways for you to decompress from the stresses of life and make the transition from stress to the simple pleasures of life. The purpose of your mental health tool box is to make the transition from your regular life to relaxing and experiencing pleasure in your personal life.

Your Mental Health Tool Box

Every day, for 10 to 15 minutes a day, you need to make a transition from your life, from making the money, paying the bills, taking care of your parents and children and pets and relationship, to get to YOUR life! Every day, you need to make the transition from the outside world, to the internal world, to your feelings, your thoughts, and yourself. Here is a guide for you on how to get there...to you!

Make a list of 10 things that you can select from that take only 15 minutes a day, more or less, to enjoy your life, to relax, to feel pleasure, and to make a transition from your position, whatever that may be, to get to your self.

I will share an example from my personal mental health tool box, on what I do to transition from therapist and writer, mother and wife, sister and aunt, "gammie" and friend, to a person. Every day after I work, before I greet my family for the night and after I see six or seven people or couples a day, I draw a hot Jacuzzi bath, with a splash of sea salt, light my unscented candles, take off my work clothes, turn on music from my expensive-but-well-worth-it radio, and sink into the bubbling jets of water. The whole world stops. My shoulders drop, my head falls back, and as I drop under the surface of the bubbling bath, my muscles all relax. All my troubles, and those from the rest of the world, including all of my clients, go away, totally leaving me and my mind free. When the water circles down the drain, I imagine all the problems circling down the drain with the water. It clears my mind, and I let go. And I simply breathe in peace. Sometimes I meditate and pray, to give me energy and let go of my fears. Then I dry myself off, put on very comfortable pajamas and go greet my family—who know not to knock on my bathroom door unless they are bleeding from the eyes! My 15 minute ritual is better than a whole bottle of Xanax.

TEN MINUTE TIP:
A TYPICAL MENTAL HEALTH TOOL BOX

1. Take a hot bath, with candles or aromatherapy, too!
2. Meditate…use a tape…it works!
3. Listen to your favorite music. Dance to it, too: by yourself, cleaning the house, or with your dog!
4. Exercise…walk, run, swim, or stretch with yoga.
5. Talk to a friend on the phone.
6. Sunbathe or moonbathe (moonbathing is a favorite of mine, where you go outside and bathe in the light of the moon and stars).
7. Get outside, even if it's driving a convertible or going for a picnic at the park or on your lunch hour.
8. Give or receive a back rub.
9. Read a good book.
10. Tune into the comedy channel and enjoy a quick round of laughter.

SEXERCISE #15

YOUR MENTAL HEALTH TOOL BOX

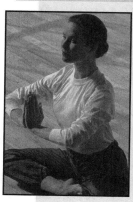

Now…make your own "TOP TEN LIST" to create your mental health tool box. Go ahead, make a new kind of list. If you can't think of anything you like to do for pleasure, steal from the list above. You'd be amazed at how many women find it very hard to come up with a list of ten things to do to nurture themselves or de-stress from the day! Put your list into your purse or wallet, so that you can refer to it every day and use it every day. Every day…take 10-15 minutes to do ONE of those things on your list, to make the transition from your life's position, to your self: mainly, to clear your mind, and to clear the way for your sexual self to come to light.

SEXUAL FANTASY AND EROTIC BEGINNINGS

For many women with low sexual desire, there are no sexual thoughts, no sexual fantasies, and they don't know where to begin to find them! As described in the last chapter, for some people sexual thoughts *follow* feelings of intimacy and closeness, meaning they don't have any sexual thoughts or fantasies until *after* they have sexual touch and begin to play sexually. If you want to OWN your sexuality and develop your own sexual identity in the way that really turns YOU on, then you will want to find out what really turns you on. Later, you can share your sexual self with a partner.

For some people, both men and women included, sex is something that happens TO THEM. In fact, life is often something that happens to them. If you are one of these people, it is as if everything comes from outside of you: You have sex when your partner wants to, you do what your partner expects you to, you do what you children need you to do for them, you complete a job at work when you are told what you are supposed to do, your family demands things from you, and so on. But if you really want to learn to love sex, realize that your sexual feelings come from *inside you*. Think about it: If you are really going to love anything—whether it is your sexuality, your car, your job, your home, but especially how to enjoy sex—then you will need to have the desire and the control and the feelings come from inside you!

Have I lost you?

Are you waiting for me to tell you what to DO to desire sex?

I will guide you...I will tell you how to get to you, but really, it is only through trial and error (and that can be the FUN part) can you figure out what you want. And here is the biggest sexual secret: You have to develop the confidence, the competence, and the comfort within yourself to experience your sexuality and to eventually share your sexual self with your partner. YOU have to develop a sexual voice, to say what you think and what you want and how you feel, if you want to be loved, to be touched, to feel good sexually. And only then will YOU feel sexual desire!

Sexual fantasy is thinking about sex and thinking about what turns you on! If you have never had a sexual thought or a sexual fantasy, I will give you a guide. First, you have to give yourself permission to have sexual fantasies. Some people think it is dirty to think about sex, or it is sexual infidelity to think about sexual scenarios that do not include their husband or current sexual partner. It is perfectly normal to have sexual thoughts and sexual fantasies. If you feel your sexual fantasies must be limited to your current sexual partner, to avoid feeling "lust" in your heart about another, then by all means…start there!

I recommend that you have a repertoire of at least your top three sexual fantasies, that you keep in reserve to use to serve only you: when you are daydreaming, when you are having sex with yourself, or when you are having sex with a partner and feel a need for more intense stimulation beyond physical stimulation, to use the mental stimulation of sexual fantasy to intensify and enhance your sexual pleasure. Yes, fantasies can intensify your sexual feelings. In fact, some women have difficulty experiencing an orgasm when they don't shift their mind from their busy life to specific sexual thoughts and scenarios in their mind during sex. Using sexual fantasies can begin sexual arousal or excitement, which can also help you to feel sexual desire! Remember: Arousal comes first, then sexual desire follows.

Think of yourself as an erotic, sexual person. Some people have negative views on sex, which can come from family or church values, or negative sexual experiences. Choose to look forward and live now, experiencing the erotic in your life as a new natural and normal behavior. Feel the experience, the touch, and the feeling first, and then allow the erotic feelings to follow.

SEXERCISE #16

SEXUAL FANTASY

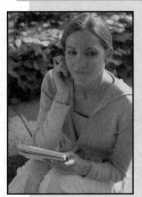

Write a paragraph or story about a sexual fantasy.

Sexual fantasies may include your past peak sexual experience, something you saw on a movie or TV, the person who you stood in line next to at the grocery store, or extensive, detailed sexual scenarios that simply turn you on! If you are like many women with low sexual desire, it is likely that you have never had a sexual thought or fantasy a day in your life. You don't know what one looks like or even if maybe you might have had one. But mostly, you think: What DO other people fantasize about?

If you feel lost, try buying a book on sexual fantasies. You could read one of Nancy Friday's books on the variety of sexual fantasies for men and for women. Her books will both amaze and, possibly, arouse you. DON'T think you need to have ALL of these sexual fantasies. In fact, some of the fantasies may turn you off, rather than turn you on. Pick out a few of your favorites, and use some parts of these to write out your sexual fantasy. You might even want to visit a website or two on erotica, and read about female sexual erotica to enhance your own personal sexual fantasies. Allow yourself to think about these fantasies while you daydream or while you enjoying sexual touch with yourself or your partner.

MIND YOUR BODY

Next comes your body, your physical sexual self. Your sexual identity requires that you mind your body. Finally, we are getting to the part where we talk about getting your body turned on! Did it seem to you as if it took forever to get here? For me, it took several months of writing, and I'm a sex therapist! For some of you, it may have taken several chapters or several years! Thank you for your patience, but I guarantee, this will be worth it!

I think it is very interesting that there are simply so many things I needed to talk to you about first, before we got to talking about turning on your body. Honestly, that is how it is in real life, too. You have so many tasks and hoops to jump through FIRST, before you get to you. Now that we're here, let's find out how to get your body tuned into your sexuality and get turned on. Remember, we're still talking about getting turned on by YOURSELF…outside the context of your relationship, which will come later.

Now, since you know we're talking about getting turned on, let's talk frankly about what makes you feel sexy and what makes your body feel sexy, too.

PLEASURE

First, let's start with pleasure in your life in general. Hedonism is often a word associated with sexual pleasure, but in reality, it is a word that means self-gratification, self-pleasure, self-satisfaction, and overall selfishness. Hedonism is usually considered a negative trait: that you are self indulgent and sinful, and usually in a sinful manner. In reality, hedonism is allowing yourself to be immersed in pleasure, including sexual pleasure. Actually, the opposite of hedonism is self-denial; the word for this is "anhedonic," which in psychology is associated with depression, or a lack of pleasure in your life.

For some people, the idea of self-pleasure is abhorrent, distasteful, and even embarrassing. It is associated with guilt: to focus on one's self and focus solely on your own pleasure. In fact, some people take a great deal of pride in being self-sacrificing and only giving to others, putting all others' needs ahead of their own.

> **If you want to want sexual pleasure, then you will need to embrace self-pleasure in your life!**

You want to embrace pleasure, not only sexually, but also in the self-indulgent ways, some of which you may have listed previously in your mental health tool kit. You want to begin to think of pleasure as a positive necessity in your life, and enjoy the pleasure of joys in every day life, including sexual pleasure. Pleasure is not just a luxury, it is a necessity that makes life worth living. Enjoy being creative with pleasure, as creativity is key in fending off depression, alongside enjoying pleasurable things in your life. In fact, here is a psychological secret:

> **The cornerstone to mental health is having something to look forward to: something pleasurable.**

TOUCH

Do you like to be touched? Do you like affection? Do you enjoy being kissed? Do you like to touch others? Do you feel comfortable with being touched? If your answer is yes and you're happy with the touch you give and receive in your life, great! But many women in low sexual frequency relationships avoid touch, which has been described repeatedly in this book. Some people like being touched, but not the way they are currently experiencing touch. The biggest problem for women is that their partners sexualize touch.

When touch is always sexualized, it feels like every opportunity for touch becomes a sexual invitation. Sometimes touch is direct groping! Most women hate groping, having their breasts or buttocks or crotch grabbed. Chapter 10 talks about the groping problem, encouraging men to stop it. It is important to directly address and talk to your partner about how you feel with touch. If you feel touch is groping or always leads to sex, talk to your partner about having touch that is nonsexual. Sexercise #9 might help you with that. Most men DO want their partners to feel safe and comfortable and pleased with their touch. Most men will listen, most of the time, when you ask them to touch you in a way that is pleasing to you. Almost all men sneak or slip, and grab once in a great while, sometimes thinking it is okay to be playful. However, if your partner won't listen to you, you might have a relationship problem, you may have a communication problem, or you may be with the wrong person. If repeated requests to change touch are ignored, seek professional help to find the root of the problem. Being comfortable with touch is very important in a loving relationship.

If you simply don't like to be touched, this matter needs to be explored more fully. Often, when people don't like touch, it is associated with one of two things: You didn't come from a "touchy-feely" home and you're just not used to it, or you experienced negative touching, including past physical or sexual abuse. In either case, it is likely that you need to make sure you are in a safe and trusting relationship, and you need to practice nonsexual touch to feel more comfortable with touch. Some people with negative pasts or experiences with touch, need to learn to become "touch tolerant." You might consider working with a massage therapist who is experienced with people who are not comfortable with touch to experience positive touch in a nonthreatening manner. Practice Sexercise #9 on nonsexual touching to grow more comfortable with touch. If you are not successful with either of these things, it is recommended that you see a professional therapist to explore your difficulty with touch.

SEXUAL TOUCH

Your sexual identity starts with YOU. You need to know what you like with sexual touch. If you know what you like and can reliably experience sexual pleasure, then you are doing well sexually. Yet many women are unable to experience sexual pleasure from sexual touch reliably, consistently, or at all. Or some women once experienced sexual pleasure, including orgasms, but they no longer have the feelings they once had.

Self-pleasuring (another word for masturbation) is often a key to discovering your sexual self and creating your sexual identity, as well as creating sexual desire. After all, if you're going to enjoy sex, YOU have to be involved in finding out exactly what you like and what you don't like. If you want to want sex, you will want to have sexual pleasure…reliably and consistently! The next section discusses how to experience self-pleasuring in different ways to discover how you like to be touched and how to bring yourself sexual pleasure, as well as different types of orgasms. If you are experienced with having orgasms, great. If not, learn to give yourself sexual pleasure, to find out what you like and don't like. Your sexual identity depends on controlling sexual feelings from the inside out, from things you do to yourself to controlling how you like to be touched. Even if you are experienced with having sexual pleasure, spend some time now to renew your sexual feelings with yourself. Take some time just for you—without anyone watching, without any imaginary clock judging how long it takes you to have an orgasm, abandoning the self-consciousness of your nakedness—by exploring sexual touch again to find out how you like to experience sexual sensations and pleasure with yourself.

If you once experienced pleasure with sexual touch, but you are currently experiencing problems with sexual arousal or excitement, then you are probably frustrated or perplexed by your sexual changes. See chapter 8 on secondary low sexual desire, to explore what may be happening for you.

ORGASMS 101: TYPES OF ORGASMS

> **Many, many women who have no sexual desire simply do not have orgasms!**

It is astounding to me how many women I have seen who are labeled as having "low sexual desire" when they have never experienced sexual pleasure, at least not with a sexual climax, either by themselves or with a partner. While it might be true that these women do have low sexual desire, it seems fairly obvious to me that if you don't get very much pleasure from sex, then you won't desire it. Who would look forward to a gourmet meal if you didn't have any taste buds to enjoy it? While pleasing one's partner and enjoying the intimacy of a sexual liaison might create some desire for sex, at least in the beginning of a relationship, when women don't experience pleasure from sex over time, they don't desire it. Sometimes the sexual problem is NOT low sexual desire, it is a lack of sexual pleasure. Most women, when they learn to have sexual pleasure, are far more interested in sharing sex with their partners.

This section teaches you how to have sexual pleasure, how to have orgasms, and even how to experience multiple orgasms more easily and reliably, so you will want to and look forward to sex and feel sexual desire! First, we'll discuss the different types of orgasms, and then explore how to have an orgasm, including how to find your "G-spot."

Generally, it is accepted that there are two different types of orgasms: clitoral and vaginal. A clitoral orgasm is a peak of sexual arousal that usually happens following touching, rubbing, stroking, or stimulation of the clitoris. The second type of orgasm is a vaginal orgasm, which results from penetration and stimulation inside of the vagina with a penis or a finger or a dildo. Yet some women have orgasms from having their nipples stimulated, or even having their toes sucked, or without ever being touched, just from fantasy[2]! Women can also have orgasms from anal sex. Obviously, the brain is very important in experiencing sexual climax, which is why some professionals believe that an orgasm is an orgasm. Regardless of the more exotic ways to experience sexual pleasure, we'll stick to the top two varieties.

CLITORAL ORGASMS

The clitoris has 9,000 nerve endings. By far, this is your best shot for a reliable orgasm. You've got several choices for stimulating your clitoris, although the creativity used in having clitoral orgasms is often amazing!

- Rubbing with your hand

- Using a shower massage
- Oral sex
- Vibrator
- Riding a horse
- Friction during intercourse
- The water jets in hot tubs/positioning under a tub faucet
- Rubbing against sheets/on a bed

By far, the most reliable method of having a FIRST orgasm, for women who have previously been unsuccessful in becoming orgasmic, is using a vibrator. I strongly recommend that women try to self-pleasure with their own hand first, but if that has been unsuccessful, get a very good vibrator. I am not talking about a hand-held, battery powered, penis-shaped piece of colored plastic. We're talking a two-speed, plug into the wall model... A real vibrator! If you haven't tried this yet, you haven't really tried a vibrator, as far as I'm concerned. Every woman should own at least one vibrator. For most women, they are worth their weight in GOLD! Two very good vibrators are the Hitachi Magic Wand, which is a classic, and the Accuvibe, which I think is even better because you can unplug it, have a battery back-up, and you don't have the cord get in your way during lovemaking.

How to Use a Vibrator...and LEARN TO LOVE SEX

The biggest barrier to using a vibrator is ordering it and using it for the first time. Many, many women I see for sex therapy tell me that they will NEVER masturbate, nor will they ever, ever use a vibrator. Ever. Yet they want to have sexual desire and learn to love sex.

- "Is there any alternative?"
- "I'll never take it out of the box!"
- "I really, really don't want to do this...EVER!"

I understand that most women are very opposed to using a vibrator. According to research surveys,[3] about 83 percent of women find the use of a vibrator "not appealing," or "not at all appealing." To be honest, in my practice, at least 1 percent of women don't end up liking using a vibrator. **But 99 percent of women like using them A LOT!**

So I strongly suggest that you try to use a vibrator for yourself: when you have some privacy, you are by yourself, no one can hear you, and no one will know! Trust me. I WANT you to want sex!

Many, many times I have worked with women resistant, reluctant, and uncomfortable to try using a vibrator or with the idea of sexual self-pleasuring. However, with a little encouragement, and sometimes because of their love and compassion for their partner and their relationship, many partners have been surprised that their partners have agreed to try a vibrator or other sexual toy.

"DOTTIE"

Dottie was 47 when she came in to see me. She had no sexual desire for her husband. She never thought of having sex with him, and they only had sex once a month or so. It wasn't that the sex was so bad: She did have orgasms with him, and she always felt good AFTER sex, but she just never thought about sex and avoided sex like the plague, being the master of sexual excuses. At first, when they married, it was the excuse of her being a virgin, then it was pregnancy, then it was the kids, then it was her job, then it was her job and stress. Suddenly, after the kids moved out...she ran out of excuses, and her husband, patient for almost 30 years, ran her right over to my office, the local neighborhood sex therapist! Dottie just couldn't get herself over the hump to start sex with her husband. She loved him, they were great friends, and she didn't understand it.

She had been brought up a strict Catholic, she was always a "good girl," and she never thought about sex.

After much discussion and cajoling, Dottie agreed to get a vibrator and try it. Despite her husband immediately ordering a Hitachi Magic Wand over the Internet for her, it sat in the closet for two months. Finally, after more encouragement, she used it. Much to her surprise...*she really enjoyed herself.* As a homework exercise, she was asked to use the vibrator, just by herself, twice a week.

In the meantime, I worked with Dottie and her husband on several different homework assignments to fan the sexual flames, including nonsexual touching, exploring sexual fantasies, learning sexual communication, improving marital intimacy, and learning sexual initiation techniques that were acceptable and even erotic. Quite frankly, nothing seemed to help improve the couple's sexual frequency.

But in the meantime, Dottie was doing the "homework" with the vibrator faithfully, twice a week every week...and sometimes more.

Even without my reminding her about it, she found herself waiting for her husband to go out, go to work, go to the hardware store, so she could get some private time, and then she would run up to her bedroom, pull out the vibrator, and enjoy sexual self-pleasuring.

With the vibrator, it was like Dottie was like a teenager again...discovering sex for herself for the very first time. Sex was on her time, when she wanted it, for how long she wanted it, and for as many orgasms as she desired, every time.

Even her orgasms became much more reliable...she could count on having two or three orgasms every time, in a short time. Heck, when her husband went to the grocery store just for milk and bread, she was squeezing in some sex time for herself. And astonishingly, she was THINKING about sex for the first time in her life. She actually found she looked forward to sex...and wanted it!

It actually took several weeks for Dottie to feel comfortable with the vibrator, and comfortable with sexual communication, before she began to share her true sexual self with her husband. But it was the use of the vibrator that she says seemed to cut through all of the other barriers of sex, and get down to her having intense sexual pleasure on her terms, before she learned to love sex, for the first time in her life!

I wish for YOU the same sexual success that Dottie and many other women have had with self-pleasuring. So here's your guide.

SEXERCISE #13

HOW TO USE A VIBRATOR

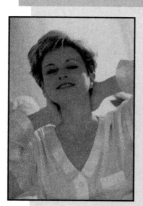

1.   Get privacy. Find a quiet time, when and where you do not feel you will be disturbed, and the noise of the vibrator will not be heard. If sound is a problem, turn on the TV in your bedroom or the radio. If you don't normally watch TV or listen to music, begin to turn them on at random times, to avoid questions and suspicion from the sex police (that is, your children, partner, or live-in parents).

2.   Get undressed and lie on the bed, leaving a little slack in the cord to move the vibrator around.

3.   Use a cloth barrier between your skin and the vibrator. At first, some women want a thick barrier, such as a pair of sweat pants or a towel. Later, you will likely feel more comfortable with a thin sheet or silk scarf. You don't have to use anything, but it can help to avoid

197

chafing or a getting pubic hair (ouch!) caught on the vibrator.

4.   Place the vibrator on low speed to start and get used to the sensations by moving it around your body, on your neck, arms, legs, and shoulders.

5.   Next, place the vibrator directly on your clitoris, located just below your pubic bone. Some women prefer to move the vibrator up and down or back and forth, while others prefer to find the right spot and leave it there.

6.   Try a variety of different pressures (soft or hard) and a combination of movements, depending on your feelings that day.

7.   Try to use the vibrator no more than 15 minutes at a time, but at least twice a week.

8.   Combine sexual fantasy (see chapter 9, if needed) with the use of the vibrator.

9.   Add in other sexual stimulation as desired, such as reading erotica or watching an adult film, during self-pleasuring.

10.   Make it a goal to share your experiences with the vibrator with your partner when you are comfortable, generally within a few months.

Hopefully, you will be successful in becoming reliably, quickly, and consistently orgasmic using a vibrator. Sometimes, it seems that the vibrator, as Dottie said, cuts through the psychological barriers to enjoying sexual responses, and lets women more easily get in touch with their sexual feelings. Clearing your mind and letting go, even using different transitions from your real life to your sexual life, can really be difficult. For some women, having direct and intense sexual stimulation from a vibrator kind of makes that transition easier, even on a bad day. Also, for some women, using a vibrator "teaches" them how to have an orgasm.

A minority of women are nonresponsive to a vibrator. In fact, some women are nonresponsive to sexual touch at all. Women describe this feeling as "being numb down there" and having no sexual sensations, despite any type of sexual stimulation. Often, this lack of sexual response is due to anxiety or self-consciousness, including body image concerns. At times, psycho–social–sexual factors combine to inhibit sexual response. If you have tried repeatedly to have direct sexual stimulation of your clitoris without success, including using fantasy or erotica for stimulation, seek professional counseling with a sex therapist.

Learn to Have An Orgasm

Many women have to "teach" themselves how to have an orgasm. Orgasms are experienced and learned over time. First one experience sexual stirrings, then learns to identify those feelings as sexual feelings, and then explores sexually find the right spots that feel good and give pleasure. For men, sex and orgasms happen to them: They wake up at 12 years old or so and they've had an orgasm! It is much more complicated for women to learn how to go with the feelings that lead them to sexual pleasure and climax. Women each need to find their own sexual pathway to pleasure, to build on those feelings with more intense stimulation, or less, in the context that turns them on (lights on/off, lingerie on/off, kissing/touching/nipples or not, fantasy or not) to create a sexual script that works for them. For some women, they find "IT"— THE right sexual moves that work, the right button, the right pathway, the only position—and they stick with it. Yet for a lot of women, if they continue exploring, they will often find multiple pathways to orgasm, including finding their G-spot (discussed below), or with female ejaculation.

"KARLY"

Karly is an African-American woman in her early thirties. She had been married to "Derrick" for three years. Karly is well-educated, a CPA and MBA, and worked in a successful law firm in town. She came in for sex therapy because she didn't have very much sexual desire. It was soon discovered that she'd never had an orgasm. Karly loved her husband, and she wanted to please him sexually, but she was getting exhausted having sex three or four times a week, after working 10 to 12 hour days on the "partner-track" in her firm.

Karly was raised in a loving, "normal middle-class" home. She had been ambitious since she was a child, and she lived at home, except for a couple of years in college, until she got married. She had dated, had had a few brief relationships, one longer-term relationship, but she had never gotten much out of sex. She had never masturbated, and it never crossed her mind, but the lack of privacy in her parent's home may have been an issue.

Basically, Karly was an overworker. She was constantly stressed out by work and rarely did anything in her life for fun. It was work, work, work, and get ahead. She wasn't very happy, although she had fun with her husband. Karly's therapy first focused on her de-stressing her life, experiencing pleasure, and learning to enjoy nonsexual touch with her husband. Next, she began to practice self-pleasuring twice a week, but she didn't want to use a vibrator.

Karly had some success in enjoying the touching exercises, and she even decided to move from a high power firm to a state government job, to decrease her work hours. And then she got pregnant, which was exciting news.

For several months, Karly came in for sessions twice a month to focus on her goals of de-stressing her life, reducing her anxiety, increasing intimacy in her marriage, and developing a sexual identity. Overall, her life satisfaction was improving, and she was developing a desire for and initiating sex once a week or so as well, but she couldn't seem to reach orgasm with her husband or on her own.

Finally, when she was seven months pregnant, Karly experienced her first orgasm, while she was using the vibrator, her

Hitachi Magic Wand. Amazingly, with her very first orgasm, Karly experienced "female ejaculation" which may occur during intense orgasm for women. A small amount (one or two tablespoons or so) of fluid squirts out of the urethra. Well, I hadn't talked to Karly about female ejaculation...and...Karly was freaked out! She thought her water broke! She threw the vibrator across the room, jumped out of bed, and called her husband:

"Derrick! I think I just had my first orgasm and I think my water broke!"

"Karly, are you having any contractions?"

"Well, no, I'm not...I just had a lot of water spray out all over the bed!"

"How much water?"

"A lot...there's a wet spot of water on the bed about six inches wide!"

Derrick laughed, and calmly replied, "But, you're not having any contractions, right?"

Karly paused and said no.

Derrick, "Karly, I think you have had female ejaculation, and that is normal and you're going to be okay!"

Karly was perfectly okay. Momentarily, she was quite freaked out thinking she was in labor, but she wasn't. Her wonderful husband came home from work and talked to her about female ejaculation, even looking it up and finding a video clip on the Internet to show her. Later, they both laughed—and so did I— about the situation. Karly didn't want to use the vibrator again while she was pregnant, but after her first orgasm, she became orgasmic through oral sex, too. Her problems with low sexual desire completely disappeared after she began to be orgasmic.

Be adventurous to find many pathways to sexual pleasure for yourself. First, figure out how your sexual wiring works through sexual self-pleasuring, then try some of the other methods, too, such as using your hand or playing with the shower massage or in a hot tub! Once you've found a sexual pathway, even only through a vibrator, be adventurous and the others will come more easily.

Expect that you will not always be successful, even with self-pleasuring. Sometimes you're just not in the right place or you're too distracted. Don't worry about it...but don't avoid returning to your pleasure!

Women who learn to self-pleasure are much more likely to discover their sexual selves, experience intimacy with themselves, and become ready to share their sexuality with a partner. Most women with low sexual desire have difficulty with the idea of masturbation. In fact, many women feel that their sexual partners should know what to do and make them have an orgasm. Many women are reluctant to take personal responsibility for their own sexuality, sometimes with a very resistant stance. The truth is, if you want someone to give you sexual pleasure, you will need to know what is sexually exciting and pleasing to you. The pathway to finding out what turns you on and excites you starts with taking control of your sexuality and owning your sexual self.

> **If your sexuality consists of "giving up" sex or having sex for someone else, in the long-run it will not be surprising if YOU DON'T HAVE ANY SEXUAL DESIRE!**

If you are not willing to discover your own sexuality and form your own sexual identity by finding out what is sexually exciting to you, unfortunately, your prognosis for changing your sexual desire is poor. If you find you have an extreme resistance to self-pleasuring (not simply a strong hesitance or dislike of the idea), and you simply cannot engage in self-exploration, you may be successful in simply working with your partner on sexual pleasuring, including the use of the vibrator, or finding your G-spot. However, most people with low sexual desire have already tried unsuccessfully to change their sexual relationship with their partner, and working on self-pleasuring alone is a needed prerequisite to partner sex. If you simply can't engage in self-pleasuring, you can work on exploring sex with your partner, and even using a vibrator with your partner. If you feel very strongly against this or embarrassed about considering the possibility, you may have a sexual aversion disorder and/or you need to seek professional help from a sex therapist.

VAGINAL ORGASMS AND YOUR G-SPOT

Only about 30 percent of women regularly have orgasms from intercourse; 30 percent of women occasionally have orgasms just from intercourse, and 30 percent of women never do (I guess the other 10 percent of women don't engage in intercourse or don't know what happens). If you are currently not having sexual pleasure from vaginal penetration, you may not be enjoying your full potential of sexual pleasure! The good news...no, the GREAT news...is that YOU can enjoy MORE sexual pleasure, by finding out, by yourself or with your sexual partner, where your G-spot is, how to stimulate it, and how to have more intense orgasms than you have ever experienced before. Most of you can learn how to do this

203

NOW! According to the "G-Spot," book, researchers found that over 90 percent of women have had success in finding their G-spot, and they learned to love sex even more[4].

And, as a woman, you might get an added bonus: You can learn to ejaculate, too! Female ejaculation is real, and it is really a different type of sexual pleasure. Some women report that vaginal orgasms are deeper, more intense "all-body" orgasmic experiences not achieved with clitoral orgasms. Plus, you might just start liking and wanting sexual intercourse, too.

The G-Spot is the area within the vagina that was described by Ernst Grafenberg and researched in the 1970s by Drs. Beverly Whipple and John Perry[5]. The researchers found a patch of skin on the upper wall of the vagina, about the size of an almond, that when touched or stimulated becomes rough in texture, like the roof of your mouth, and swells in size and becomes "spongy" feeling. Some women have a sensation of having to urinate when their G-spot is stimulated. Don't let that sensation stop you! When it is stimulated, women sometimes expel a fluid from their urethra, and ejaculate, just as men do when they have orgasms. Just as with men, this ejaculate is not urine, even though both fluids are expelled from the urethra.

Find the spot, find the way, and you may learn to love sex…you might never have to be convinced you to want sex again! And with a vibrator or the Hitachi Magic Wand, with the special attachments, you can discover your G-spot on your own.

SEXERCISE #14

HOW TO FIND YOUR G-SPOT

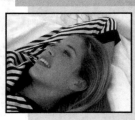

1. Get in the mood. The G-spot gets engorged with blood and swells when you're sexually aroused, so it will help your sexual responsiveness if you're turned on. *Read some erotica or fantasize.* Use your vibrator or self-pleasure first, to get aroused, but don't have an orgasm.

2. Locate the G-spot. It is located on the top side of your

vagina, or on the upper side where you belly button is located. Insert a finger inside your vagina, reaching upwards, but not as far as your cervix, the hard round mound in the back of your vagina. You should feel a slightly ridged area on the upper wall, about two or three inches inside your vagina.

3.   Feel the G-spot. The texture feels noticeably different from the typically smooth walls of the vagina, when it is excited. When not aroused, it is hard to find because it will be smoother, like the rest of your vagina. Since it expands, it will vary in size, depending on your level of sexual excitement at the time.

4.   Stimulate the G-spot by pressing on the spot, and stroke it by using a "come hither" motion with your fingers. You can also use a sexual toy, such as the G-spot attachment on the Hitachi Magic Wand, the longer blue "crooked" attachment. It can be much easier to stimulate your G-spot with a vibrator or attachment.

5.   Squeeze your PC muscle, like you are doing kegels, or making yourself stop urinating in the middle of a flow. A well-toned PC muscle will help increase your sexual sensitivity and your ability to ejaculate. Feel the muscles bearing down on your finger or vibrator.

6.   Apply pressure to the toy so that you can experiment with the amount of friction you prefer against your G spot. Don't be afraid to apply firm pressure. Try a variety of movements: back and forth, circular, a vigorous thrusting, or with or without vibrations.

7.   You'll know you're hitting the spot as you feel tingly sensations and you will often feel the urge to urinate. This is when a lot of women hold back, fearful they will urinate. FEAR NOT: You will not release urine; the response is incompatible with female ejaculation, as it is when men ejaculate.

8.   Let go. Continued your G-spot stimulation, and add in clitoral stimulation as well, if you'd like. You may or may not ejaculate, but ejaculation is perfectly normal.

9.   If you don't orgasm, try using clitoral stimulation at the same time. If you aren't successful, try again later: It can take several practice sessions before you notice any success. Good luck!

SHARING YOUR SEXUAL SELF

Practice self-pleasuring on your own until you feel very comfortable with sexual pleasure and you have developed confidence with giving yourself orgasms. If you haven't learned how to have G-spot orgasms on your own, don't worry. Sometimes it is easier to find and stimulate your G-spot with the assistance of a partner—and it can be a fun sexual activity for a couple, too!

Deciding when to share your sexual self varies greatly among people, from a few weeks before you feel so excited you want to share your discoveries, to several months before you will feel sexual excitement and confidence with your new sexual identity and sexual self. Remember, most guys have been doing this for YEARS before they share their sexuality with a partner! Just be sure you feel comfortable with your sexual self first, then move on to creating sexual intimacy…for TWO!

Moving on to sharing your new sexual self with your partner is a challenge for many women, while it comes naturally and is very fun for others. For some people, the suggestion that you share what you have learned about your body and what you like is very scary. Many women feel very self-conscious about their bodies in general, but even more so with the idea of *showing* their partner exactly what they like sexually. Ideally, a woman can explore her body until she is comfortable with bringing herself pleasure, and then show her partner how she self-stimulates by masturbating in front of him. Some women are absolutely horrified by this idea, and never show their partners what they do or like! Some of these women work very hard during sex to move their pelvis around to follow their partners hand, mouth, or sexual parts to feel pleasure, rather than using their voice to say what they would like, or simply showing them.

While sharing may seem really hard to do, it might be important to know that *every* man I have ever worked with in therapy has been very open to their partner sharing their likes and dislikes with them, especially by showing them exactly how they like to be sexually stimulated. Men crave information and direction to help them help you enjoy pleasure. Men also do better with visual instructions than verbal suggestions. Remember that almost every couple is very successful when they try it, and they feel closer afterwards. I strongly encourage you to try to do this with your partner, so they can know what to do to please you. To help you get started, here are a couple of tips.

TEN MINUTE TIP FOR SHARING SELF-PLEASURING

- First, simply talk to your partner to see if he or she would like to talk about what you like sexually. Next, talk to your partner about if they would like to be with you, while you sexually pleasure yourself. 99.9 percent of men will be excited about it and will encourage you.
- Second, ask your partner to be present the first time, but to close their eyes. Just get comfortable with having them near you, in the same room.
- Third, ask your partner NOT to watch you as if you were a TV. Ask him to hold you and caress you, which would seem more natural for love-making.
- Fourth, if you are using your hand, let him put his hand on you, then you put your hand on top of his, to guide him in the best motion or position or pressure to show him how you like to be touched. If you're using a vibrator, hold it together.

Sharing your sexual self with your partner can be intimidating and scary at first, but when you open yourself up to your partner and feel encouragement, support, and love, you will feel closer and more intimate with your partner. You can experience sexual desire again (or for the first time) by introducing sexual touch and sharing sexual behaviors first, then allowing sexual desire to follow. Understanding this new approach to sex will allow many lower-desire partners to experience sexual feelings, sexual pleasure, sexual enpowerment, and a new sexual relationship with their partners.

THE HIGHER-DESIRE WOMAN

If you are the partner with higher desire, know that you really are not alone! Since nearly 15 percent of men have low sexual desire, millions of women like you are in relationships or marriages with men who have little interest in sex. As a woman, you can feel very isolated, since all of the jokes about couples not having sex revolve around women who won't "give it up" to their husbands, and men who complain about their sexually disinterested wives. Society accepts that men "never get enough sex," while women are accused of intentionally holding out on men sexually. Men are supposed to want more sex than women, right? So women fear that if all men want is sex and their husband doesn't want them for sex, there must be something wrong with them. Sadly, women who suffer in low sex relationships feel embarrassed to reveal that they want sex more than their partners. Women that suffer in sexless marriages have suffered silently.

The tide is turning. More women are coming forward, publicly sharing their frustrations with their partners' lower sexual desire. In fact, the media is now reporting stories about sexless marriages, in which the men have lower desire. The following was found on AOL News in August, 2006.

"SEX-STARVED WIFE ASKS POLICE FOR HELP!"[6]

Police in the German city of Aaschen received an unusual call for help late Wednesday when a woman telephoned to complain her husband was not fulfilling his sexual obligations.

After the couple had been sleeping in separate beds for several months without intimate contact, the 44-year-old woman woke the husband, 45, in the middle of the night and demanded he satisfy her needs, police spokesman, Paul Kemen said Thursday.

When her advances were refused, a row broke out and she called the police and asked them to intervene, he added.

"Sex-starved" may not be how women would like to be characterized, but the problem of sexless marriages in which women are the higher-desire partners is getting recognition. However, there is still little research on marriages and relationships with men who have low sexual desire. Many men are reluctant to come forth for treatment, most likely fearing a stigma of not being "a real man" if they doesn't desire sex. As with men who are in marriages with low or no sex, women feel very sad, isolated, frustrated, and angry about the lack of sexual closeness and physical intimacy.

Until recently, women tended to fall into two distinct categories as the higher-desire partner in a sexless marriage: sexually ashamed or the sexual castrator. In the past several years, another category of higher-desire women has appeared: the sexually defiant.

THE SEXUALLY ASHAMED

The first category is, sadly, women who are married to men with low sexual desire and blame themselves for their lack of sexual frequency, feeling unattractive or sexually inadequate. Sexually ashamed women make false assumptions about why their partners do not want to have sex. These women assume their husbands don't love them, that they aren't attractive or sexy enough, they are too fat, or don't have big enough breasts, and perhaps because of their inadequacy, their husbands are having affairs. Some women fear their husbands are gay, and sometimes they are right, but they don't talk about it. One client I knew had a breast augmentation because she thought her husband wasn't attracted to her before she found out he was attracted to men. These women suffer in silence. Often, they cannot get their husbands to go to therapy. They might even feel too embarrassed for their husbands to make them come to therapy, where they fear they will be humiliated or ridiculed for not wanting sex. Many eventually lose their greater sense of sexual energy and accept a sexless marriage.

THE SEXUAL CASTRATOR

Some higher-desire women relate more to the anger or sexual frustration or sense of betrayal that men who have higher-desire than their partner feel. Some women take on similar roles as men who become coercive and badgerers when their partners do not want to have sex (see chapter 3). However, the reason men don't want to have sex in the first place, starting the sexual power struggle, is usually different than women's. Some men become sexually distant from their wives because they feel so nagged and belittled, emotionally domineered and verbally assaulted, that it is as if they are emotionally sexually castrated by their partners. Some men feel their partners are so rude and mean that these sensitive men lose their ability to sexually function with their wives. After highly anxious and negative sexual encounters, these men continue to perform poorly sexually, resulting in further emotional assaults and greater sexual distance. Men who have unresolved anger and avoid conflict resolutions often develop sexual dysfunctions, such as low sexual desire and erectile dysfunction. In truth, women can also be sexually coercive and sexually hostile, and it fuels the sexual power struggle described in chapter 2. When sexual conflicts reach this level of tension in the relationship, professional attention is often needed.

THE SEXUALLY DEFIANT

This woman tends to be more secure about her own sexuality. This woman tends to feel very confident about her sexuality, has fully claimed her sexual identity, enjoys healthy sexual relationships, and enjoys emotionally close relationships, as well. This woman may have a greater sexual energy than her monogamous partner, but she is not threatened, nor threatening, about her sexuality. This woman seeks to have a healthy, active sex life. The sexual defiant woman says, "I'm going to have sex, whether it is with you, or by myself. I will work with you to overcome your sexual problems and any relationship problems I am causing to solve our problem. I am not willing to be a nonsexual person." She may seek medical help for her partner who has erectile problems or rapid ejaculation. She may openly disclose her masturbation behaviors, or she may choose to end a relationship, over time. This woman seems to be empowered by economic independence and psychologically healthy feelings about herself and her life. She is not willing to be sexually dissatisfied, but she is neither hostile, nor passive.

The Sexual Solution

Women with higher desires need to read chapter 10 on causes of lower desire in men, which rarely has to do with men's feelings of love or attraction for their partners. In fact, men have very similar reasons for not desiring sex as women, such as relationship conflicts, depression, and sexual problems. While women experience the problem of sexual pain and avoid sex, men experience premature ejaculation and erectile dysfunction and fear poor sexual performance. In practice, distance in a couple's emotional relationship due to unresolved conflicts or resentments is the most common cause for low sexual desire, after medical and sexual problems in men. In addition, couples tend to lose the habits of romantic and sexual relationships as they get busy with their lives, work, and families.

As with men, women need to remember that sex is a basic instinct, a biological need, and a normal human drive. Almost every healthy human feels a need for sex; you are wired for sex from birth, and there's not a thing wrong with you for wanting to have sex and make love with your partner. It is also very important to feel wanted by your partner. You want to be wanted as much as you desire your partner, right? Yet if you are going to be successful in having sexual change, you have to start by finding the true cause of low sexual desire and work toward a true change starting with your relationship.

As with couples where the man has higher sexual desire, couples with women with higher sexual desire need to work as a team to become sexual partners. See chapter 10, on taking on a role as a sexual partner, and the section "A Guide to Sexual Partnership." Couples with discrepant desire can also work together on the Ten

Minute Sexual Solution. First, begin with sexual communication, then developing emotionally intimacy, followed by physical intimacy with touch, and then sexual touch. In order to work the Ten Minute Sexual Solution, higher- and lower-desire men and women need to seek to understand the true causes of low sexual desire, rather than reacting to each other out of false assumptions, jumping to irrational conclusions, and behaving as if these causes were real, such as thinking their partner does not love or want them. Each couple needs to start with reassurance of their love, and a commitment to work the Ten Minute Sexual Solution together.

Higher-desire women and lower-desire partners often can bridge their sexual compatibility gap with maintenance sex. Sexual synchronicity works best if the focus of sexual accommodation is not exclusively on sexual intercourse, but on sexual pleasuring, as discussed in chapter 7. The next chapter includes a section for lower-desire male partners, as well as higher-desire male partners that women with higher-desire may also relate.

CHAPTER

10

Ten Minutes a Day: For Men

Do you feel saddened, frustrated, or betrayed sexually in your relationship? Do you feel like your desire for sex is ignored in your relationship? Does it seem to you like you have to jump through 100 hoops for your partner just to get a kiss, a hug, a flash of naked flesh, or maybe, on a very good day, to make love? Does it seem like the window of sexual opportunity in your relationship is barely open a crack? If you are married, does it seem like as soon as you said, "I do," she said "I don't" when it came to sex?

If so, this chapter will help you reclaim and begin to discover your sexual power as a man. Much of this chapter is aimed at the higher-desire man, the vast majority of men, yet many higher-desire women will relate to it, too. The end of the chapter speaks to men with lower desire.

A man was asked, "How many minutes a day would you be willing to devote to sexuality?" He answered, "All day!"

Surprised? Does it seem like all men would be willing to devote all day, every day, any day to sex? Well, the truth is…yes and no!

While up to 15 percent of men suffer from low sexual desire, the majority of men are in relationships where the man has a stronger sexual drive and he feels dissatisfied, angry, or perplexed about low sexual frequency. The truth is that many men feel disheartened and even betrayed by their partners, especially their wives, due to the lack of sex in their relationships.

So what does this anger and frustration look like for the typical higher-desire/lower-desire couple? For most couples who live together, even couples in long-term marriages, if a whole week goes by and you haven't had sex all weekend long (not counting "that time of the month") there's a big problem for the person who really wants sex. Ever hopeful, the weekend begins with the excitement, anticipation, and hopefulness of looking forward to *the weekend*, but it can transform into anger and resentment, as described below.

THE SEXLESS WEEKEND

As a busy couple, you didn't have time for sex all week long, and you are looking forward to lovemaking on the weekend! Friday night arrives, and maybe you barely share a stiff hug when you greet each other at the end of the work week. You share a peck of a kiss goodnight before you fall into bed, but it's okay, because you were tired from work and a long week. Saturday morning comes, and you wake up with a morning woody that you're hoping to use. Sadly, you realize that your wife has leapt out of bed, mind bogglingly at 7 A.M., and is already knee deep in plastic gloves and bleach, with no plans to return to the bedroom. Morning comes and goes, yet Saturday night you're still hoping, and you start trying to get something sexual started. You start dropping hints, making sexual gestures, trying to do everything just perfectly, crossing off every chore on your list, trying not to make her mad, so you can crack open that window of sexual opportunity for some

Saturday night sex. Saturday night comes and goes, and you're disappointed (or worse yet, sexually frustrated and rejected!) when nothing happens. Why?

The long unanswered questions begin to creep in as Sunday arrives, with the last vestiges of sexual optimism gleaming in the eye of the person with the higher sexual desire. A bright, hopeful, high browed look turns into a bitter stare as another weekend closes without any sex. When you go to bed, you shut your eyes and suck in air through your teeth, restless with sexual agitation. Your back turns aggressively away from your partner, while no body parts make contact, and you try desperately to fall off to sleep. Monday morning hits and the anger and resentment are carried to work, along with your briefcase and palm pilot. A lot of people ask themselves, on the way to work Monday morning...What the hell happened last weekend? Or last month? Or for the last year? How many weekends have to go by, without any sex? If the average person wants to have sex at least a couple of times a week, why are we having problems enjoying lovemaking even ONCE on a normal weekend? Why did we have another sexless weekend?

WHAT HAPPENED TO YOUR SEX LIFE?

Most people stay together or get married because they want each other, they can't stand being apart from each other, they love each other, they're attracted to one another, and they have had really hot sex or fantastic lovemaking...at least in the beginning of their relationship. Even partners who were both virgins when they married often report they did "everything but intercourse" before the wedding night, and they *struggled* to keep their hands off each other when they dated.

Gradually, you don't touch anymore. Now you struggle to keep your hands off each other, not because you can't stop touching each other, but because you can't touch each other without a strange awkwardness that separates you or leads to a major fight. She doesn't kiss or touch because of fear that it will lead to a turn-on or a come-on and sex, which she is avoiding. You can't touch her because she'll push your hand away (and we're not talking about groping here), or because she'll tense up, or even act as if your hand isn't there. She avoids you. This is the one that hurts the most. She stays in a different room. She goes to bed earlier or later. She moves around you when she walks by, instead of toward you. She dresses so that her clothing covers every possible exposure of her skin, even in bed at night. She sleeps with your child, and you sleep alone. Or you sleep with a child between you. Nobody kisses each other passionately, because you just don't do that anymore unless you're having sex, if then. On a good day, or just a normal day, you peck each other on the lips or the cheek, while saying goodbye for the day or goodnight when it's right and she gives you two pats on the back, on the head, or on the hand. Count them: It's the two pat finish. Two pats, and you know it's over. It hurts to feel so alone. There is no place so alone, as when you're alone in a marriage.

MEN FEEL BETRAYED IN SEXLESS MARRIAGES

Every week, I have women come into my sex therapy office and sit on my couch and tell me that they have no interest in sex. Sadly, sometimes tragically, this is your marriage or your committed relationship. Truthfully, you need to realize that many people don't want to feel this way, to have no desire for sex, and they are often coming to therapy to find out why and to try to fix the problem. I am very happy to help them and to help you, too, because I want both of you to enjoy the physical pleasure of sharing your love together. Yet secretly, at times I feel sorrow watching your struggle in a sexless relationship, especially when you love your partner so much, feel so much attraction, even when you *know* they love you. Usually, they do love you, but they don't know how to feel sexual desire, and it has nothing to do with you.

As you sit in my waiting room, or on the couch across from me in my office, I can see there's no playfulness in your physical affection. No wet kisses, no furtive fondling. Yet you often hold hands and comfort each other and wipe each other's tears. On the one hand, I feel sad, but on the other, I feel hope knowing that there really is a chance for most couples in a sexless relationship.

It's so important for you to know that most women don't choose to lose their sexual desire. Most women did not know they have low sexual desire before they got married. Yes, a few women admit they do not like sex, and they only had sex when you were dating because "that's what you do when you're dating," and then they stopped having sex after you had children. Men feel betrayed that they are now "trapped" in a sexless marriage. Even then, it is important for you to know that often it is because many women were simply not raised to be sexually open or healthy in our society, and they have not experienced their full sexuality yet. Sometimes it is because they made a vow of chastity that they saved for you. Other times it is because their chastity was robbed from them through sexual assault, rape, or mistreatment by men who came before you. Sometimes there are relationship problems that both of you know you need to resolve and that both of you most likely share responsibility for changing. In the meantime, while you are both sexually suffering, it isn't fair! But the good news is that there is really hope, and your attitude toward change can make or break your marriage.

When sex becomes a problem, it accounts for the majority of marital dissatisfaction...from 50 to 70 percent of the marital problems! On the other hand, for couples who are happy with their marriages and sex life, they feel that only 15 to 20 percent of their marital satisfaction comes from sex.[1] In other words, if you are having a sexual problem, it dominates the marriage, but if you're doing okay, people tend to take it for granted as a part of a satisfactory relationship.

This is not at all surprising to me. Think about food. If you are hungry, you are thinking about food all the time: "I'm starving, I want to eat, where can I get a meal, when will we eat next?" The mind is on food, food, food…it's obsessed! On the other hand, if you're getting plenty to eat, you don't think about food very much at all…hmmm, maybe only 15 percent of the time! If your hunger drive is met, you don't think about it, but if it is NOT met, you will think about it all the time, try to meet it, and it will dominate your life. The same phenomenon happens with your sex drive!

That is why the lower-desire partner in a relationship often views the higher-desire partner as "perverted" or "a sex addict" or "never satisfied with sex!" Because most of the time, the higher-desire partner is simply hungry all the time because they feel sex-starved!

So I'm going to try to help you have more sex and make more love. Sex is a basic instinct, a biological need, and a normal human drive. Almost every healthy human feels a need for sex; you are wired for sex from birth, and there's not a thing wrong with you for wanting to have sex AND make love with your wife or lover. Don't get me wrong, if you're like the typical man I see on my couch every day, you are NOT just interested in having sex! You want to be close to your partner, you want to touch her, feel her, even listen to her, but mostly:

You want to be wanted!

You want to be desired and wanted by your lover, your wife, your bride, your partner, as much as you desire her, right?

THE HIGHER-DESIRE MAN: TYPES OF SEXUALLY FRUSTRATED MEN

If you are reading this, it is likely that your attempts to convince your partner to have more sex with you have failed. In different ways, people get sexually desperate. Men try to change their situation, their relationship, and their marriage. Generally, men fall into one of the following three categories, when they are faced with a sexless marriage.

THE SEX SUPERVISOR

This man tries to become a sexual supervisor of his relationship. He takes on his role as the manager of his sexual relationship, similar to a business manager. He counts how many times he has had sex and categorizes what kind of sex he and his partner have had, including sexual intercourse and oral sex (or how long it's been). Sometimes he becomes very attentive to the sexual problem and works to solve the situation. He tries to talk to his partner like a parent to a child, to tell her what she needs to do and change to be a better sexual partner. He may read magazine articles or books, search the Internet, or even find a therapist, to suggest new ways to solve the problem. His role as supervisor is on again, off again, moving in on the project, then getting distracted with other projects in his home, work, or life. Like the role of a supervisor in one's job, he can be loved and/or feared, but when he gets his eye on you, you feel like you're being scrutinized, and you get nervous. The supervisor might buy this book, looking to solve the problem.

THE SEXUAL BULLY

The sexual bully uses sexual coercion (an act of emotional force or threat) and verbal badgering until his partner agrees to have sex. Often, the lower-desire partner controls sex by not wanting, refusing, or avoiding sex (see chapter 2). The higher-desire partner can become a sexual bully when he reverts to coercion or verbal badgering to reverse the control of sex. Sometimes the coercion or use of force is mild or subtle: A sexually rejected man gets into a bad mood or broods until his wife finally agrees to have sex so that he'll stop pouting or being grouchy. In an extreme form, a man may make threats to his partner to make them have sex, including withholding money, threatening to have an affair, or threatening a break-up or divorce. Read chapter 2 on sexual power struggles to understand and break the cycle of sexual coercion.

THE SEXUALLY DEFEATED

This man is often more emotionally sensitive than the other two types of men. This man does not want to force his wife or partner into doing anything she doesn't want to do. He often feels emotionally rejected by his wife by getting turned down for sex. Tired and hurt from being rejected for sex, he stops initiating sex and waits for his wife to initiate sex, when she is willing. As a result, he rarely has sex, if he has a partner with low sexual desire, especially if his partner does not like to initiate sex. This man wishes he could stop being attracted to his wife, or even wanting sex, because his attraction and desire cause him emotional pain. Sometimes this man is a conflict avoider, who would do anything to avoid a fight, especially about sex.

Can you identify your type? As a sex supervisor or sexual bully, if you are the one who is taking responsibility to solve your sexual problems and trying to try convince your partner have more sex with you, I'm going to let you know right now that you can't do it alone, and you will continue to fail. You can bully your partner in a subtle or extreme way, or chase your partner around the house with a book or threats for the next 25 years, but you can't make her read it or do anything in it to change. Your behavior will only result in her having more resentment, which creates sexual pressure, less sexual desire, and less satisfying sex. And if you remain sexually defeated, your sexual relationship won't change, either!

Your job as the sex supervisor needs to end. Your behavior as a sexually bully has to end or it could end your marriage, too. Your role as the sexually defeated will not change your sexual relationship, either. So what do you do to solve your sexual problem? You need to take on a new role as a man.

THE SEXUAL PARTNER

The sexual partner is, first and foremost, on an equal level with his partner. The sexual partner takes on a role as a supporter to understand what might be happening with his partner, and to become a part of a partnership, because she needs you as much as you need her. While it is true that your partner is going to at least want to want change, if you change how you act toward her, you have a chance to change your marriage. You can try out this new role, in conjunction with new solutions for your sexual problem and relationship found within *The Ten Minute Sexual Solution*, to begin in a different way, a better way, a beautiful way to sharing a physically loving relationship.

A GUIDE TO SEXUAL PARTNERSHIP

Your first barrier to being successful in solving your sexual problem is acknowledging, as a couple, that you have a problem, and to create a sexual partnership. The first homework exercise in chapter 2 talks about talking to your partner about reading this book, and the second sexercise encourages making a sexual commitment. But what are you going to do if you disagree about having a problem? Sometimes people with less sexual desire know they have a problem, because they know they don't feel a desire for sex or enjoy it, and they recognize that this isn't normal, especially if they once felt sexual desire but don't anymore. Yet sometimes people who have low sexual desire don't think they have a problem. Some people make it clear that that they don't think it is THEIR problem, or they blame their partner: "I don't have a problem, YOU do! You're oversexed (or perverted or a sex addict), so YOU deal it!" Whether the lower-desire partner sees that it is her problem or your problem, as a couple you do have A PROBLEM with sex.

Sometimes in long-term relationships, after arguments have failed to solve the problem, sex becomes an unspoken topic that you avoid. In reality, long-term avoidance can make it seem like there isn't a problem, because it is such a relief to stop fighting about sex. As with the sexually defeated, sometimes the higher-desire partner stops initiating sex, but they can still be very resentful and dissatisfied sexually. Over time, the lower-desire partner can feel like everything is okay, because sexual demands and fights decrease, so, for her, it might seem like there's no problem.

Whether you are arguing about sex, or you are avoiding talking about it, whether one of you admits it or not:

> **If one of you is sexually dissatisfied, you have a sexual problem AS A COUPLE. You both have to agree on this fact to solve the problem.**

Some people think it takes two people to change. No—it only takes one person to put change into motion. Think about it like this: When you come home from work, could you change the mood of the household, simply by how YOU act? If you walked in the door, slammed it shut, threw your keys down on the kitchen counter and stomped upstairs, silently brooding or even ranting and raving, wouldn't you change and determine the mood for the entire night? But if you went home tonight, greeted your partner a smile, a bouquet of flowers, brought home a completely prepared dinner, then offered to help the kids with their homework and baths (or take care of the pets), how differently would your night proceed? It would change! One person can set into motion a course of actions to create feelings that can affect your entire household and relationship! The same concept can be applied to your intimate and sexual life.

As a couple, I want you to have an opportunity to work the Ten Minute Sexual Solution, as a sexual partnership. As a team, you can restart intimacy and communication, and sex, even maintenance sex, for busy couples! The Ten Minute Sexual Solution cuts through some of the psychological barriers, resentments, and excuses for sex, and makes it possible for couples to experience more frequent sexual activity. Since this chapter is just for men, we are going focus on what you can do as a man, as an individual, to set into motion changes that will make the Ten Minute Sexual Solution become a successful program of change for you!

> **NOW, I'm going to tell you some things you probably won't like about WHY you have a sexless relationship... that have to do with YOU!**

WHY MEN HAVE A SEXLESS RELATIONSHIP

It is unlikely that all of your sexual problems are your partner's fault. It is possible, but unlikely. The last two chapters have addressed your partner's problems with low sexual desire, focusing on why she might now want to be having sex, and how she can make changes to share a different marital and sexual relationship. In some relationships, one person truly has an individual problem with having low sexual desire that has absolutely nothing to do with you. If this is the case, then it is likely that this section will not apply to you. Yet in most relationships and marriages, a man must take a look at himself, to find out why he has a sexless relationship. In this section, you will not find the cheerful, scientific explanation or professional version of sex therapy that you might be expecting to solve your problem of a sexless marriage. Throughout this book, you will find professional sex therapy advice on improving your relationship and sex life, but this section tells the naked truth of why *some* men simply aren't getting laid.

The naked truth, having worked with thousands of couples for over 20 years, is this:

> **The number one reason why your partner won't have sex with you is because they're angry with YOU!**

Quite frankly, many partners are pissed off with their partners, and feel powerless to change it, whether they realize it or not. People continually get angry over little and big things that YOU do to mess up, and they lose sexual interest. For example, a wife doesn't want you sexually when she's mad at you. A wife doesn't want to make love when she is so busy doing "everything" around the house that she doesn't have the energy left to give anything to you. While some women call this fatigue, it usually is accompanied by anger that they don't get enough help. Chapter 6 discusses at length how to learn to fight, so you can start making love. You might have thought it strange that a book on sex spent an entire chapter talking about how to fight right and how to resolve conflicts in order to improve your sex life. The beginning of the chapter said: Anger poisons a sexual relationship. Anger is not an aphrodisiac. What the chapter did NOT say is how powerful anger is in creating a sexless marriage. The most important thing to remember if you have a low sexual frequency marriage or relationship is that women FIRST need to feel emotionally close, emotionally connected to their partners, and free of emotional conflicts before they feel sexual desire. If a woman is mad, even over little things, she will not want to have sex!

If your partner was once attracted to you, emotionally and sexually, she'll want you more when she is not as frustrated, irritated, exhausted, and mad! More importantly, if your partner admires and respects you and appreciates many things that you do, she will feel more attracted to you, and make love to you more often. Or at least she will want to please you sexually (through maintenance sex or sexual accommodation or even oral sex), even if she is not sexually interested, if you are pleasing her in other ways, outside of the bedroom.

> **Start pleasing your partner outside the bedroom, and she want to please you more inside the bedroom!**

Chapter 5 was all about creating intimacy outside of the bedroom. Creating an intimate bond is essential to having a foundation for lovemaking. Working on the Ten Minute Sexual Solution to create more intimacy will help you. However, as a man, you need to know what to do on a daily basis, so you don't make your partner mad at you, which can reverse all of the progress you can make when working on the sexercises.

SEXUAL EXPECTATIONS

When you were dating, or let's say when you were 20 years old, all you had to do was look cute or "hot" and have a car for a girl to be interested in you. If you weren't particularly good looking, all you had to do was be nice to a girl. That's it! That's all it took! You looked good, listened a little, talked nicely, and you got a date! Right? Well those days are over, aren't they? Let's take a quantum leap into the reality of marriage and the expectations of life and long-term relationships! If you see yourself as an ideal man, who almost always pleases his partner, almost always takes her advice, does what she asks, completes household tasks without asking, helps out with the kids even more than your fair share, maintains the house, treats your parents and family with kindness and respect, takes responsibility for your own business and personal needs without leaving them for someone else to do, and brings home a paycheck that allows your family to live comfortably, and your partner is still not interested in a sexual relationship with you, then the problem may not lie with you or be in your power to change.

However, if you are not a saint (and who is?) and your partner complains and nags or simply seems to "bitch for no reason" then you need to start listening to her! What is she complaining about? What is she unhappy about? You need to find out exactly why "she's bitching all the time!" Believe it or not, women do not wake up in the morning and think, "Hmm…what can I find to bitch about today?" Most likely, your partner wakes up thinking about how to have a good day, and runs into problem after problem that she blames on you. She gets angry, eventually solves the problem herself, and then feels resentful of you because you didn't do what you "were supposed to do!" By the end of the day, why should she do anything for you, especially have sex, when she had to take care of so many things all day that *you were supposed to take care of?* Suddenly, there is no energy or desire left for sex, for you! Think about it: What has your partner TOLD you she is angry about?

TEN MINUTE TIP: EXPECTATIONS FROM WOMEN

The bottom line is that many women lose sexual desire because they are angry with their partners, and/or they are exhausted from taking care of more than their share of household chores, even if you don't know it. Plus, women have resentments from problems in the past or long-standing disagreements. Resentments may come from unresolved conflicts in many parts of your relationship, such as where you live, how many children you have, your relationship with your mother, addictions, money, affairs, or other sexual matters. If you want to get to the root of your sexless marriage, take a look at yourself, find out what the expectations are for your relationship, and revisit self-examination.

> **Most importantly, search for the reason why you are not emotionally connected.**

SELF-EXAMINATION

Look back at chapter 6, under the heading of self-examination. If you haven't already done so, answer the question: "Would you want to be married to you?" Do you have shortcomings? Try talking directly to your partner, admitting your faults, and making apologies as necessary, then make a commitment for change. Start building trust by keeping promises. Certainly, major life problems, such as addictions, chronic work problems, medical problems, or affairs, will require professional help. If you have a major problem, get the help you need, stop delaying it, and make a commitment to change that will work toward gaining back marital trust and loving feelings.

Sometimes men think that providing a paycheck and money is their contribution to the household and that should pretty much cover most things. First of all, it's highly likely that your partner also brings home a paycheck, but maybe also has a second job of being a homemaker and mother, too. You may think you contribute and show your love by sharing your earnings, but this is simply not going to be enough, even if you're a multi-millionaire. What happens outside the household can be irrelevant when it comes to sexual feelings inside the house. Make sure that you do not create resentments over unmet household expectations that can create a wedge between the two of you.

Besides money, what do you do to contribute to your relationship that makes your life better? Is it fair? For example, yard work is seasonal work, and it doesn't require daily maintenance. "I take care of the outside, and she takes care of the inside" is never a fair deal, and most men know it! Ask your wife or partner what kind of things she resents and how you can help to change those feelings of resentment.

In the long-run, when partners feel more appreciated they will appreciate you more, too. What do you do that makes it worth your partner's while to be a part of your life? If you can't think of three things off the top of your head, read below about doing kind and caring things. Eventually, your behavior outside the bedroom may change her behavior inside the bedroom.

KINDNESS AND FORGIVENESS

A minister once told me that he thought kindness was the most important ingredient in a good marriage. Kindness is an important ingredient in feeling close to someone and creating goodwill. If you're looking for sexual goodwill, practice kindness. Many years ago, when I first got married, in my early twenties, I thought, "Gee, I had better be nicer to my husband since we're going to be together for a long, long time." That may sound kind of silly, like why wouldn't I be nice to him anyway? But for some reason, after going through that marriage ceremony and making a lifelong commitment, I suddenly thought that I should act more kindly. It's a good idea to put credits into your marriage's or relationship's emotional bank.

> **Kindness is an investment in kindness.**

Unless you're in a relationship with a self-centered, narcissistic person who will just take advantage of you anyway, generally, the more you give, the more you get back. Kindness in thought, word, and deed go a long way toward preserving love and relationships. People in happy marriages report experiencing five good things to one bad thing, a 5:1 ratio. Certainly, there are going to be times when you will take some debits, some withdrawals out of that emotional bank, right? But do the good things to balance out with the bad days. Most couples I see in sex therapy report ratios of 1:1 on the good/bad scale or lower! If you haven't done so already, put some kindness and forgiveness in the emotional bank called your relationship.

Kindness can include simple acts of caring like bringing your lover a cup of coffee in the morning or taking the garbage out without being asked. It can mean giving compliments and receiving them graciously. Think of trying to do two caring things for her every day, things that take only a minute or 10 to do. Do what your partner thinks is caring, not how you like being cared for. For example, my husband brings the newspaper in and puts it on the kitchen table for me almost every morning. If he is really running late, he throws it in the front door. He knows I love to read the paper every morning with my coffee or tea. He doesn't read the paper; he does this to show me he is thinking about me and he cares about me, even though I'm usually still sleeping when he leaves. I can walk downstairs in my pajamas, and I don't have to get dressed to get the morning paper, which is especially nice in the cold weather. I love it! It is a way for him to say "I love you," and it takes him one minute. Caring behaviors might include a sending a text message, saving the last piece of chocolate cake, or remembering to encourage someone about a big meeting that day. If you don't know what to do…if you are clueless…don't wait for the clue fairy: ASK! "What would you like for me to do for you, for 10 minutes a day that would make you feel cared for?" It takes so little and it means so much, just once or twice a day.

Kindness also means being loving when somebody's made a mistake. It means that you don't make a big deal over little mistakes, like burning a chicken dinner or ruining a shirt in the laundry. It means giving your partner a hug when they total your new car instead of getting mad, because you're happy they're alive! It means giving your partner a hug when she didn't get a promotion or he loses his job, instead of questioning/criticizing her immediately, such as "What did you do wrong that you got fired?" Part of kindness is being forgiving. Being forgiving is an important gift of love, especially when someone's wrong. It counts in little ways like being understanding when a check bounces, but it is essential in healing pain from marital wounds, such as infidelity and addictions. Thoughtfulness, consideration, and forgiveness are kind acts of love.

SEXERCISE #17

CARING BEHAVIORS

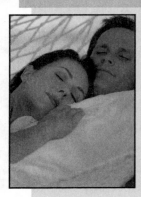

Think of two things to do for your partner every day, to act caring toward them. These caring behaviors might only take a minute or two to do, but they can create emotional warmth and let your partner know you are thinking about them and care. Examples include calling them to say you're thinking of them or love them, sending a card or writing a note, or completing a dreaded household chore without being asked. If you can't think of anything to do, ask you partner, "What would you like me to do for you that shows you I care about you?"

If all of these suggestions fail, ask friends or relatives in your life, who know your partner, what they think the problem might be. You don't have to talk to them specifically about sex, but ask them how your partner feels about you, what they say about you, and what their complaints are, to find out what is wrong. Also, ask them what you might do to be pleasing and kind to your partner: What does she like, what flowers make her smile, where does she shop? Find out, just as if you were dating and newly interested in her.

If you work on being kind and considerate, giving and forgiving, and are working on your own personal faults, but none of it makes a difference in your partner's feelings or attentive behaviors toward you, seek professional help from a sex therapist, social worker, psychologist, or counselor. As a marriage and sex therapist, I find that most men are really great guys, but they are often clueless when it comes to pleasing their partners. Sometimes their partners are very difficult to please, though! Most men really want to do the right things to make their partners happy, and their children's lives happy, while providing for their families. Most men need a little guidance to find out how to do the right things to make their relationships better and a gentle nudge and reminder to keep the caring behaviors going. Get started and see what you can do right now, on your own, to create change in your relationship or marriage.

MEN WITH LOW SEXUAL DESIRE

Men who are dissatisfied with sex in their relationships tend to fall into two major categories.

1. Men who have low sexual desire, who often have their partners chasing after them, feeling dissatisfied that they are not getting enough sex

2. Men who constantly complain that they are simply not getting enough sex.

The majority of men are dissatisfied because they aren't getting enough sex, yet 15 percent of men, millions of men, experience a lack of sexual desire. These men hide behind an invisible wall of secrecy and, often, shame or guilt. Being a man who doesn't want sex is like being a boy who doesn't like baseball. You're an outcast amidst the crowd, where it's safer to suffer in silence and secrecy than expose your true self. Young boys suffer in right field, facing ridicule and dreading the southpaw who comes up to bat. Men who have low sexual desire suffer alone and in relationships, dreading exposure when they have to come up to bat. Ultimately, because of their lack of interest, their overall performance suffers, and they fail again.

Amazingly, men with low and high desire have one major characteristic in common. Both men with high and low sexual desire have mental distortions about intimacy, a problem that is strikingly similar! Men who have low sexual drives sometimes avoid dating and sex, but when in relationships and marriages, they drive their partners crazy with not wanting sex, resigning themselves to an inability to seek intimacy. And men who constantly complain about not getting enough sex do not understand how intimacy is the answer to getting more sex! Both groups of men need to learn about being intimate with themselves and with their partners. Men in general, but specifically men with sexual problems, need to work on the intimacy aspects of their relationships. Chapters 5 and 6 both address intimacy problems and solutions, including communication and intimacy outside the bedroom. Working the exercises in the Ten Minute Sexual Solution helps men with intimacy problems, regardless of their relationship and sexual problems.

Low sexual desire for men is a complex sexual problem, as it is with women. Intimacy problems alone are often rooted in complex psycho-social factors. Past physical, sexual, and relationship traumas can affect desire, but sometimes it is simply unresolved conflicts and anger in relationships. Low sexual desire in men has only recently been seriously addressed by writers, researchers, and the media, so new information and treatment interventions is likely forthcoming. The following are common factors currently known regarding inhibited sexual desire in men.

COMMON REASONS FOR LOW SEXUAL DESIRE FOR MEN

- Depression
- Obesity
- Stress and overworking
- Medical problems, such as low testosterone; however, contrary to popular belief, testosterone is an uncommon cause of low sexual desire for men. Other medical problems, such as diabetes, can cause sexual dysfunction, which doesn't lower desire to have sex, but increases sexual avoidance
- Avoiding problems with sexual performance
- Alcoholism
- Social anxiety disorders (fear of social scrutiny)
- Lack of attraction to your partner.
- If are you gay, and have not yet come to terms with it, or are in a "Save Yourself From Homosexuality Marriage"
- Relationship/marital problems

- Conflict avoidance in the relationship, which leads to resentments
- Sexual pressure from women

Most of the common reasons for low sexual desire in men are self-explanatory. However, a few of the more complex reasons for low sexual desire will be described in detail below.

Conflict Avoidance in Men

Among the common reasons for low sexual desire is avoiding conflicts the relationship. Conflict avoidance is broad category that includes avoiding dealing with emotional distress or disagreements in relationships, which leads to emotional and sexual shut downs. One reason for conflict avoidance is unresolved conflicts or built up resentments in a relationship, which is addressed in chapter 6. Another typical scenario seen in sex therapy is a relationship in which a man feels emotionally dominated by his partner, and he has learned from his past relationships or in the current relationship that it is better to shut up and agree, than to speak up and start a fight, or at least it seems that way. In response, this man stops talking and stops starting sex, or he stops saying why he feels emotionally hurt and stops asking for what he wants sexually and his sex drive stops, cold. This is a form of sexual self-defensiveness and sexual passive-aggressiveness described in chapter 2. See chapter 9 discussing the sexual castrator, to get a portrait of some women who are in the role of sexual bullies.

Fear of Sexual Performance

Another common reason many men have low sexual desire is because they avoid sex when they have concerns over sexual performance. Some men do not actually have lower sexual desire; in fact, they do desire sex. However, they don't initiate sex or they avoid sex because of their fear of sexual failure. Some men have erection or ejaculation problems (usually too fast), and they don't want to deal with it themselves or with their partners. One-third of men have problems with premature ejaculation, and most men have problems with erectile dysfunction occasionally and increasing with age and medical problems.

Rather than discuss sexual problems with their partners, and even their doctors, many men avoid both sex and relationships that might lead to sex. Many men feel too ashamed to talk about their problem, so they avoid sex completely. Some men need only to experience one or two or even three times where "things just did-n't work" before they give up on having sex. For some couples, one or two negative sexual situations create a great deal of anxiety, or even sexual rejection or a sexual fight. After a few of these horribly embarrassing or anxiety-provoking events, some men emotionally shut down and avoid sex, rather than talk about it or deal with it. Recently, I had a man in therapy that didn't date for 10 years because he had a problem with premature ejaculation. He had been embarrassed and somewhat humiliated by two sexual failures, and he simply stopped dating to avoid a repeat performance. Fortunately, with medication and therapy, this man began dating and enjoying a sexual relationship.

Almost all men have problems with erections at some time in their life. Actually, a man's age coincides almost perfectly with the percentage of men with erection problems. This means that at 40, 40 percent of men have mild to severe erection problems; at age 70, nearly 70 percent of men have erection problems, and so on.[2] In truth, most (80 percent) of men's problems with erections are attrib-uted to medical problems, at least initially. After experiencing a "sex-ual failure," men have anxiety over sexual performance, which caus-es a mixture of physical and psychological sexual problems. Less often, erection problems are attributed to psychological factors, such as stress, anxiety, and relationship problems. Some men get Viagra (or Levitra or Cialis) for erection problems, and often it solves the sex-ual problems, but sometimes it doesn't and then sex shuts down

TEN MINUTE SEX TIP FOR MEN: ON ERECTION PERFECTION

ALL men, of EVERY age, have problems with erections from time to time. Maybe it's the sexual situation, the fact that you're tired, you drank too much, or your sexual timing was off. Every couple has sexual "failures." Part of sex is a numbers game: If you have great sex 9 out of 10 times, then you have great sex! If 1 out of 10 times, the sexual situation just doesn't work, accept it! It's normal! NO couple has fantastic, peak sexual experiences every single time, at all ages! Don't seek erection perfection: Learn to laugh at yourselves and enjoy sexual intimacy and the pleasure of sexual touch, rather than focusing on one sexual performance to measure who you are as a man or as a couple.

again. Some men who have only rare or occasional sexual problems use drugs such as Cialis to have "erection insurance." Regardless of the source of the problem, if men have erectile dysfunction and it is untreated by medication or sex therapy, they will often shut down sexually and have low sexual desire. Even if they desire sex, they may avoid it, which is not really a desire problem, but a performance anxiety problem. Most partners think that you don't desire sex or them, when in fact, you are simply avoiding sexual performance failures.

Men often have difficulty with intimate communication with their partners, especially regarding their sexual functioning. Some men turn to a pill prematurely to deal with erection or ejaculation problems. It is strongly recommended that you men work on sexual communication exercises and increasing intimacy, particularly emotional intimacy in your relationship, but also physical intimacy. As men get older, their needs for touch, especially direct sexual touch for arousal and having erections, increase. Men need to learn and practice talking comfortably with their partners, developing a sexual voice for themselves and what they would like as far as physical affection and touching. Some men, who are not "sissies," would like to experience a connection with their lover, rather than simply supplying an erection for sex. For men with intimacy and communication problems, work on the sexercises for just 10 minutes a day in chapters 5 and 6. If you have little or no success in changing your relationship or how you feel, I recommend that you practice the art of self-pleasuring or masturbation as described below in Sexercise #18.

> **If you want to have sexual intimacy with another person, first you need to learn to have sexual intimacy with yourself.**

SEXERCISE #18

MASTURBATION FOR MEN

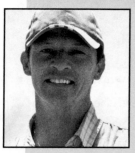

While most men have experienced masturbation, if you would like to experience the art of self-pleasuring and learn a more holistic, body-centered way of enjoying sexual pleasure, especially if you are currently not experiencing sexual desire in your life, I strongly recommend that you read *The Multi-Orgasmic Man: How Any Man Can Experience Multiple Orgasms and Dramatically Enhance His Sexual Relationship* by Mantak Chia and Douglas Abrams.[3] This is a fantastic book for men that really can't be duplicated here or improved upon. The concepts are detailed, yet simple to understand and follow. You will learn a holistic approach to whole body sexuality for men, how to tune in to your body more, and how to have more intense sexual pleasure, including how to have multiple orgasms! I recommend this book for all men, not only men with lower sexual desire. Micheal Castleman's book, *Great Sex*,[4] is an incredible book for men on increasing sexual pleasure and has an awesome chapter on premature ejaculation.

Whether you are a man who is experiencing low sexual desire, or you are a man with a higher desire in your relationship, *The Ten Minute Sexual Solution* was written to help you and help your partner simply enjoy more sex! You may need to go through several steps to learn sexual communication, how to fight right, improve your intimacy, and learn a few sexual scripts for maintenance sex, but the whole idea is simply for you to put more love into lovemaking, and do it more often. I truly believe that if you follow these steps, you have a very good chance of success and can change your sex life now! I wish for you that your partner will participate in reading this book and that you can enjoy sharing homework assignments together, embracing both of your sexualities, so you can enjoy a happier, more fulfilling sex life together!

A Closing Note from Dr. Darcy

My hope for ALL of you is that the Ten Minute Sexual Solution is successful in creating a sexual solution for both you and your partner. Differences in sexual desire, low sexual frequency, interrupted intimacy, and low sexual desire affect both individuals and couples in overwhelming ways.

My wish is for you to work together as a couple by beginning to simply become closer as a couple first, then open up your mind, body, and souls to a new level of sexual connection.

My challenge to you is to work on the relationship conflicts that inhibit emotional and sexual intimacy, by learning how to fight right. Taking the self-examination, doing a personal inventory, and working the steps of fighting right, while remembering not to fight to win, is tough work. Resolving conflicts, making agreements and keeping them, and dissolving resentments is what I call the real "work" of relationships and marriages. Learning to fight right, to stop arguing and start making love, is painful, but necessary to make a passionate sexual relationship possible.

My gift to you is to present in one book a sex therapy program to guide you to a new level of emotional intimacy, sexual communication, and sexual pleasure that will result in your making love more often.

The Ten Minute Sexual Solution is a powerful guide, packed with many sexual secrets, ten minute tips, sexercises, professional guidance, and real sexual solutions. This book is intended for many couples that cannot afford sex therapy, do not have access to sex therapy, or would simply like to work on improving their marriage or relationship in a private, self-directed approach. For some couples, gaining knowledge and using only a few techniques in this book will profoundly change their sexual identities and sexual life. For other couples, this book will be only a beginning for change, helping you to identify your strengths and growth areas, and to empower you with knowledge and skills that will set you on a life long journey of sexual happiness.

I wish you all the sexual success in the world. Good luck!

Resources

CHAPTER 1

1. Davis, J., Smith, T., Marsden, P. (2003). *General Social Survey: 1972-2002: Cumulative Codebook.* Chicago: NORC.
2. Laumann E., Paik, A., Rosen R.. (1999). Sexual dysfunction in the United States: Prevalence and predictors. *Journal of the American Medical Association.* 1999; 281: 537-544.
3. Laumann, E., Gagnon, J., Michael, R., Michaels, S. (1994). *The social organization of sexuality.* Chicago: University of Chicago Press.

CHAPTER 2

1. Laumann, E., Gagnon, J., Michael, R., Michaels, S. (1994). *The social organization of sexuality.* Chicago: University of Chicago Press.
2. Laumann E., Paik, A., Rosen R.. (1999). Sexual dysfunction in the United States: Prevalence and predictors. *Journal of the American Medical Association.* 1999; 281: 537-544.

3. American Psychiatric Association. (2000). *Diagnostic and statistical manual of mental disorders DSM-IV-TR.* Fourth Edition, Text Revision. Washington, D.C.: American Psychiatric Publishing.

4. Foley, S., Kope, S.A., Sugrue, D.P. (2002). *Sex matters for women: A complete guide to taking care of our sexual self.* New York: The Guilford Press.

CHAPTER 3

1. Harris, R. (1994). *It's Perfectly Normal: Changing bodies, growing up, sex, and sexual health.* Cambridge, Massachusetts: Candlewick Press.

2. Luadzers, D. (2006). *Virgin sex for girls: A no-regrets guide to safe and healthy sex.* New York: Hatherleigh Press.

3. Luadzers, D. (2006). *Virgin sex for guys: A no-regrets guide to safe and healthy sex.* New York: Hatherleigh Press.

CHAPTER 5

1. Michael, R., Gagnon, J., Laumann, E., Kalota, G. (1994). *Sex in America.* Boston : Little, Brown.

CHAPTER 7

1. Laumann, E., Gagnon, J., Michael, R., Michaels, S. (1994). *The social organization of sexuality.* Chicago: University of Chicago Press.

CHAPTER 8

1. Laumann, E., Gagnon, J., Michael, R., Michaels, S. (1994). *The social organization of sexuality.* Chicago: University of Chicago Press.

2. Laumann E., Paik, A., Rosen R.. (1999). Sexual dysfunction in the United States: Prevalence and predictors. *Journal of the American Medical Association.* 1999; 281: 537–544.

3. Masters, W.H., Johnson, V.E. (1966). *Human sexual response.* Boston: Little, Brown.

CHAPTER 9

1. Laumann, E., Gagnon, J., Michael, R., Michaels, S. (1994). *The social organization of sexuality.* Chicago: University of Chicago Press.
2. Whipple, B., Ogden, G., & Komisaruk, B.R. (1992). Physiological correlates of imagery induced orgasm in women. *Archives of Sexual Behavior,* 21 (2):121–133.
3. Laumann, E., Gagnon, J., Michael, R., Michaels, S. (1994). *The social organization of sexuality.* Chicago: University of Chicago Press.
4. Ladas, A., Whipple, B., Perry, J. (1982) *The G Spot: And other discoveries about human sexuality.* New York: Dell Publishing.
5. Whipple, B., Perry, J., Ladas, A. (2005). *The G Spot: And Other Discoveries about Human Sexuality.* New York: Owl Books.
6. Reuters. (2006). Sex-Starved Wife Asks Police For Help. <http://news.aol.com/topnews/articles/_a/sex-starved-wifeaskspoliceforhelp/n20060803080709990005?cid=936>

CHAPTER 10

1. McCarthy, B. & McCarthy, E. (2003). *Rekindling Desire: A Step-by-Step Program to help low-sex and no-sex marriages.* New York: Brunner-Routledge.
2. Feldman, H., Goldstein, I., Hatzichristou, D., Krane, R., Mckinlay, J.. (1994). Impotence and its medical and psychosocial correlates: Results of the Massachusetts Male Aging Study. *Journal of Urology.* 151: 54–61.
3. Chia, M., Abrams, D.. (1997). *The Multi-Orgasmic Man: Sexual Secrets Every Man Should Know.* San Francisco: Harper.

4. Castleman, M. (2004). *Great Sex: A Man's Guide to the Secret Principles of Total-Body Sex.* Ashford: Rodale Press.

ADDITIONAL RESOURCES

1. Lew, M. (2004). *Victims no longer: The classic guide for men recovering from sexual child abuse.* Second Edition. New York: Harper Books.
2. Maltz, W. (1991). *The sexual healing journey.* New York: Harper-Collins.
3. Masters, W.H., Johnson, V.E. (1970). *Human sexual inadequacy.* New York: Little, Brown.
4. Smith, T. (2003). *American Sexual Behavior: Trends, Socio-Demographic Differences and Risk Behavior.* University of Chicago: National Opinion Research Center, GSS topical report No. 25.

Index

A

accepting, 71
adult-centered family, 49–50
adult time, making time for, 49–51
(Almost) Famous Ten Minute
    Maintenance Sex Solutions, 157
anger, role of, 108, 135
attraction, role of, 42–43
avoiding the blame game, 129

B

badgering, sexual, 25–26
being judgmental and blaming, 70
betrayed in sexless marriages, feeling,
    216–218

C

caring behaviors, 230
circle of attraction, 43–44
clitoral orgasms, 193–194

coercion, sexual, 25–26
compromising, 127–128
conflict avoidance in men, 233
couples and low sexual desire, 41–42
creating sexual synchronicity, 137–138
creating sexual transitions, 167, 168
creating your sexual identity, 179–180
cycle of sexual power struggles, 26–27

D

desire, role of sexual desire, 8–9
developing a sexual voice, 79
did you turn off your sexual switch?,
    173–175
differing sexual desires, over, 21
Dr. Darcy's formula for successful sex-
    ual communication, 66–68
Dr. Darcy's Intimacy quiz, 92–93
Dr. Darcy's Ten Rules for How to
    Fight Right, 113
dyspareunia, 36

E

emotional connections, fading of, 1
endometriosis, 38
expectations, sexual, 225-226

F

fantasies, sexual, 186-187
fear of sexual performance, 233-237
Fietsam apology, 125-126
fight right, learn to fight
    admit when you are wrong, 123
    anger, role of, 108, 135
    avoiding the blame game, 129
    brainstorm real solutions for real
        problems, 127
    call a time-out and cool off, 117-
        118
    compromising, 127-128
    cooling off, 119-120
    do finish a fight, 118
    do not play the divorce card, 122-
        123
    Dr. Darcy's Ten Rules for How to
        Fight Right, 113
    expectations, role of, 131-132
    Fietsam apology, 125-126
    fighting to win, 110, 121-122
    learn to say "I'm sorry," 124-125
    negotiable and nonnegotiable
        matters, 130-131
    no abuse, 113-115
    resentments, 129
    self-examination: your look in the
        mirror, 132-133, 134
    silent violence, 120-121
    solve the real problem, 126-127
    take turns being right, 127-128
    take turns raising kids, 128-129
    take turns with anger, 115-117

    taking responsibility in your rela-
        tionship, 133
    unmet expectations, 132
    unresolved conflict, 109
fighting to win, 110, 121-122
friendship and intimacy, role of, 94-95

G

G-spot, 193, 203-204
getting off track, 61-64

H

higher-desire man: types of sexually
    frustrated men, 219-221
higher-desire partner, 14-17
higher-desire woman, 207-209
how to find your G-spot, 204
how to use a vibrator, 197
hypoactive sexual desire disorder, 34

I

inhibited sexual desire (ISD), 32
initiation, sexual, 83-84
intimacy
    creating a solid foundation of, 47,
        105-107
    the importance of, 91-93
    types of, 93-94
Intimacy exercise: sexual turn-
    ons/turn-offs, 97
Intimacy over time exercise, 107

K

kindness and forgiveness, role of, 228-
    231
kissing, avoiding, 103
kissing, importance of passionate, 101-
    102

L

low sexual arousal or excitement, 39-40

low sexual desire
attraction, role of, 42-43
causes and types of, 32-34
circle of attraction, 43-44
classifications of low sexual desire, 34
couples and low sexual desire, 41-42
definition of, 34-35
hypoactive sexual desire disorder, 34
inhibited sexual desire (ISD), 32
low sexual arousal or excitement, 39-40
medical causes for sexual desire and arousal problems, 40-41
primary low sexual desire, 34
secondary low sexual desire, 34
sexual aversion, 40
sexual pain, 35-39
situational low sexual desire, 34
lower-desire partner, 9-14
lubrication, 37-38

M

maintenance sex, 7-8, 48, 53-54
(Almost) Famous Ten Minute Maintenance Sex Solutions, 157
creating sexual synchronicity, 137-138
definition of, 138-140
five steps to maintenance sex, 155-156
overview, 136
sexual mapping, 140-144
making a commitment to change, 82

making sex a priority: special communication, 81-83
marriage, importance of a great, 89-92
masturbation, 152-154, 236
medical causes for sexual desire and arousal problems, 40-41
men and discovering your sexual power
betrayed in sexless marriages, feeling, 216-218
conflict avoidance in men, 233
expectations, sexual, 225-226
fear of sexual performance, 233-237
guide to sexual partnership, 221-223
higher-desire man: types of sexually frustrated men, 219-221
kindness and forgiveness, role of, 228-231
men with low sexual desire, 231-233
overview, 213-214
self-examination, 227-228
sex supervisor, the, 219
sexless relationships, and, 223-225
sexual bully, the, 219-220
sexual partner, the, 221-222
sexually defeated, the, 220-221
what happened to your sex life, 215-216
Mental Health Tool Box, 185
mental health tool box, 183-185

N

negotiable and nonnegotiable matters, 130-131
new approach to creating sexual desire, 159-162, 166-167

nonsexual touching (NST), 104
normal sexual desire, 9
NST: A touching exercise, 104

O

one minute kissing exercise, 102
orgasms, 192-194, 199-203

P

passive-aggressive behaviors, 28-29
"penis problem," 102-103
physical sexual self, 188-189
physical touch and sexual desire, 162-
  166
playing together and intimacy, 98-
  100, 99-100
pleasure, role of, 189-190
power struggles, sexual
  cycle of sexual power struggles,
    26-27
  differing sexual desires, over, 21
  fears in a sexless relationship, 24-
    25
  overview, 20-21
  sexual badgering, 25-26
  sexual coercion, 25-26, 27
  sexual differences, 21-24
  solutions to, 31-32
  truth about power struggles, 30-
    31
primary low sexual desire, 34, 169-
  172
priorities and The List, 182-183
priority of sex in your life, 4

R

resentments, 129
roommates rather than lovers, 3

S

secondary low sexual desire, 34, 172-
  173
self-defense, sexual, 28
self-examination, 132-133, 134, 227-
  228
sex and affection, 100-101
sex supervisor, the, 219
sex talk, the, 74
sexercises, 56-59
  sexercise #17—Caring behaviors,
    230
  sexercise #12—Creating sexual
    transitions, 168
  sexercise #3—Developing a sexu-
    al voice, 79
  sexercise #14—How to find your
    G-spot, 204
  sexercise #13—How to use a
    vibrator, 197
  sexercise #6—Intimacy exercise:
    sexual turn-ons/turn-offs, 97
  sexercise #10—Intimacy over
    time exercise, 107
  sexercise #4—Making a commit-
    ment to change, 82
  sexercise #18—Masturbation for
    men, 236
  sexercise #9—NST: A touching
    exercise, 104
  sexercise #7—Playing together,
    99-100
  sexercise #16—Sexual Fantasy,
    188
  sexercise #5—Sexual initiation,
    87
  sexercise #2—Sexual language, 75
  sexercise #8—The one minute
    kissing exercise, 102
  sexercise #1—The sex talk, 74

sexercise #15—Your Mental Health Tool Box, 185

sexercise #11—Your sexual cycle, 147

sexless mind, the, 180

sexless relationships, 1, 4-5, 24-25, 223-225

sexpectations, 147-149

sexual accommodation, 149-152, 149-153

sexual aversion, 40

sexual avoidance, 61-64

sexual badgering, 25-26

sexual bully, the, 219-220

sexual castrator, the, 209-210

sexual coercion, 25-26, 27

sexual communication

  intimacy, and, 6

  sexual rules, and the, 80-81

sexual communication, secrets of accepting, 71

  basic communication tips, 68-69

  being judgmental and blaming, 70

  Dr. Darcy's formula for successful sexual communication, 66-68

  initiation, sexual, 83-84

  making sex a priority: special communication, 81-83

  the sex talk, 72, 73

  sexual communication and the sexual rules, 80-81

  sexual Pandora's box, 72-73

  spontaneous sex, the myth of, 84-87

  talking tips, 69-70

  your sexual voice, 74-79

sexual conflicts, 8

sexual control, 30

sexual cycle, 147

sexual cycles, 146

sexual desire, create, 8-9, 48

  creating sexual transitions, 167-168

  did you turn off your sexual switch?, 173-175

  new approach to creating sexual desire, 159-162, 166-167

  overview, 158

  physical touch and sexual desire, 162-166

  sexual intimacy with yourself, 175-176

  sexual touching paradox, 162

  situational sexual desire problems, 174-175

  your sexual self: primary low sexual desire, 169-172

  your sexual self: secondary low sexual desire, 172-173

sexual differences, 21-24

sexual fantasy, 188

sexual frustration, dealing with, 144-145

Sexual initiation, 87

sexual intimacy with yourself, 175-176, 180

Sexual language, 75

sexual mapping, 140-144

sexual pain, 35-39

sexual Pandora's box, 72-73

sexual partner, the, 221-222

sexual position transition, 182

sexual self: primary low sexual desire, 169-172

sexual self: secondary low sexual desire, 172-173

sexual solution, the, 211-212

sexual touch, 191-192

sexual touching paradox, 162
sexually ashamed, the, 209
sexually defeated, the, 220-221
sexually defiant, the, 210-211
sexually transmitted infections, 38
sharing your sexual self, 205-208
silent violence, 120-121
situational low sexual desire, 34
situational sexual desire problems,
    174-175
spontaneous sex, the myth of, 84-87
synchronicity, creating sexual, 137-138

T

taking responsibility in your relation-
    ship, 133
talking tips, 69-70
touch, role of, 190-191
turning on your mind, 181-182

U

unmet expectations, 132
unresolved conflict, 109
urethra infections, 28

V

vaginal orgasms, 203-204
vaginismus, 36, 38
vibrators, using, 194-199
voice, your sexual, 74-79

W

women and discovering your sexual
    power
    clitoral orgasms, 193-194
    creating your sexual identity, 179-
        180
    fantasies, sexual, 186-187
    G-spot, 193, 203-204

higher-desire woman, 207-209
mental health tool box, 183-185
orgasms, 192-194, 199-203
physical sexual self, 188-189
pleasure, role of, 189-190
priorities and The List, 182-183
sexless mind, the, 180
sexual castrator, the, 209-210
sexual intimacy with yourself, 180
sexual position transition, 182
sexual solution, the, 211-212
sexual touch, 191-192
sexually ashamed, the, 209
sexually defiant, the, 210-211
sharing your sexual self, 205-207
touch, role of, 190-191
turning on your mind, 181-182
vaginal orgasms, 203-204
vibrators, using, 194-199